GUT HEALTH

Nourish Your Microbiome for Optimal Wellness

SARA BLAIR

© COPYRIGHT 2024

All right reserved.

INTRODUCTION

In the intricate web of our body's biological orchestra, there exists a powerhouse often overlooked but vital to our overall well-being—the gut. Defined not only by its role in digestion but as a complex ecosystem of microorganisms, the gut holds the key to a revolution in our understanding of health. The significance of gut health extends far beyond mere stomach comfort; it permeates into every facet of our existence.

As the gateway to the body's internal universe, the gut is home to a vast and diverse community of bacteria, viruses, and fungi collectively known as the gut microbiome. This bustling metropolis, residing in the depths of our digestive system, orchestrates a symphony of functions that extend well beyond the breakdown of food. It serves as a linchpin for our immune system, a hub for nutrient absorption, and even influences our mental well-being through the mysterious gut-brain connection.

The gut microbiome, often referred to as our "second brain," is a dynamic and adaptable system that responds to the choices we make daily. Diet, lifestyle, and environmental factors intricately shape this microscopic community, dictating whether it thrives or falls into disarray. Hence, the choices we make regarding our gut health carry profound implications for our physical and mental resilience.

In recent years, a paradigm shift has occurred—a Gut Health Revolution. Researchers and health enthusiasts alike are delving into the intricacies of this microbial world, uncovering the profound impact it has on our day-to-day lives. This revolution is not a fleeting trend but a scientific awakening, a realization that the gut is not merely a passive player in the background of our health narrative but a central protagonist in the epic tale of our well-being.

Join us on a journey through the labyrinth of the gut microbiome—a journey that transcends traditional views of health and wellness. As we unravel the secrets of gut health, we will explore the symbiotic dance between our bodies and these microscopic allies, the factors that influence their harmony, and the pivotal role they play in maintaining balance within us.

Fasten your seatbelts, for we are about to embark on a voyage into the heart of the Gut Health Revolution—a revolution that promises not just digestive comfort but a holistic transformation of our understanding of health itself.

CHAPTER ONE

Gut health refers to the overall well-being and optimal functioning of the gastrointestinal tract, a complex system responsible for the digestion and absorption of nutrients, as well as playing a crucial role in various physiological processes. The term encompasses the balance and harmony of the gut microbiome, a diverse community of microorganisms that inhabit the digestive system, including bacteria, viruses, and fungi.

A healthy gut is characterized by the effective digestion of food, absorption of nutrients, and the maintenance of a balanced and diverse microbiome. This balance is essential for the proper functioning of the immune system, metabolic processes, and the prevention of various health issues.

Gut health is influenced by a combination of factors, including diet, lifestyle, environmental exposures, and genetic predispositions. Diets rich in fiber, prebiotics, and probiotics, along with adequate hydration, contribute to a thriving gut environment. Conversely, factors such as a diet high in processed foods, overuse of antibiotics, chronic stress, and lack of physical activity can negatively impact gut health.

Understanding and prioritizing gut health is increasingly recognized as a key component of overall wellness, with emerging research highlighting its connections to not only digestive health but also to immune function, mental health, and the prevention of various chronic diseases. As a result, the concept of gut health has gained prominence in both medical and popular discourse, leading to a "Gut Health Revolution" that emphasizes the importance of fostering and maintaining a healthy gut for optimal well-being.

SIGNIFICANCE OF GUT HEALTH

The significance of gut health extends far beyond its role in digestion; it permeates into virtually every aspect of our overall well-being. The gastrointestinal tract, often referred to as the "second brain," is a complex and dynamic system that plays a pivotal role in maintaining homeostasis within the body. Here are some key aspects that underscore the significance of gut health:

Digestive Function:

• Nutrient Absorption: The gut is responsible for breaking down food into its basic components, facilitating the absorption of essential nutrients such as vitamins, minerals, and amino acids. A healthy gut ensures efficient nutrient absorption, supporting overall bodily functions.

Gut Microbiome and Immune System:

• Microbial Balance: The gut is home to a vast array of microorganisms collectively known as the gut microbiome. This diverse ecosystem interacts with the immune system, influencing its development and response to pathogens. A well-balanced microbiome is crucial for a robust immune defense.

Metabolic Health:

• Regulation of Metabolism: The gut microbiome plays a role in metabolic processes, including energy extraction from food and the regulation of metabolism. Imbalances in the gut microbiome have been linked to conditions such as obesity and metabolic syndrome.

Mental Health and the Gut-Brain Axis:

• Gut-Brain Connection: Emerging research has unveiled a bidirectional communication system between the gut and the brain known as the gut-brain axis. The gut can influence mental health, mood, and cognitive function, with disruptions in gut health potentially contributing to conditions like anxiety and depression.

Inflammatory Response:

• Inflammation Regulation: A healthy gut helps regulate inflammation. Chronic inflammation in the gut is associated with various diseases, including inflammatory bowel diseases (IBD), and has implications for systemic inflammation linked to conditions such as cardiovascular disease.

Detoxification:

• Elimination of Waste: The gut is responsible for the elimination of waste and toxins from the body. A well-functioning gut ensures efficient and timely removal of waste, preventing the accumulation of harmful substances.

• Barrier Function: The lining of the gut acts as a physical barrier, preventing harmful substances and pathogens from entering the bloodstream. A healthy gut lining is crucial for maintaining this barrier function and protecting against infections.

Vitamin Synthesis:

• Production of Vitamins: Some bacteria in the gut contribute to the synthesis of certain vitamins, such as B vitamins and vitamin K. These vitamins play essential roles in various physiological processes.

Recognizing the significance of gut health has led to a paradigm shift in healthcare, with a growing emphasis on promoting a healthy gut environment to prevent and manage various health conditions. The Gut Health Revolution reflects a broader understanding of the interconnectedness of gut health with overall physical and mental well-being.

OVERVIEW OF THE GUT MICROBIOME

The gut microbiome is a vast and dynamic community of microorganisms residing in the gastrointestinal tract, playing a fundamental role in maintaining the health and balance of the human body. Comprising bacteria, viruses, fungi, and other microbes, the gut microbiome forms a complex ecosystem that interacts with the body in multifaceted ways. Here's an overview of the key aspects of the gut microbiome:

• Diversity of Microorganisms: The gut microbiome is incredibly diverse, with trillions of microorganisms representing thousands of different species. This diversity contributes to the microbiome's resilience and ability to adapt to various environmental factors.

• Location and Composition: The majority of the gut microbiome resides in the large intestine, particularly the colon. The composition of the microbiome can vary along the length of the gastrointestinal tract, with distinct microbial communities in the stomach, small intestine, and colon.

• Bacterial Dominance: Bacteria make up the majority of the gut microbiome. The two predominant bacterial phyla are Bacteroidetes and Firmicutes, though other phyla contribute to the overall diversity. Each individual's microbiome is unique, influenced by factors such as genetics, diet, and environment.

• Digestion and Nutrient Absorption: Certain microbes aid in the breakdown of complex carbohydrates and fibers, facilitating digestion and the extraction of nutrients from food.

• Metabolism: The gut microbiome contributes to the metabolism of certain compounds, influencing energy balance and storage.

• Immune System Support: The microbiome plays a crucial role in the development and regulation of the immune system, helping to defend against pathogens.

Gut-Brain Axis:

The gut microbiome communicates with the central nervous system through the gut-brain axis, a bidirectional signaling pathway. This interaction has implications for mental health, mood, and cognitive function.

Influence of Diet:

Diet is a major factor shaping the composition and function of the gut microbiome. High-fiber diets, rich in fruits and vegetables, promote the growth of beneficial bacteria. Conversely, diets high in processed foods may contribute to an imbalance in the microbiome.

Stability and Resilience:

A healthy gut microbiome is characterized by stability and resilience. This resilience allows the microbiome to recover after disturbances, such as antibiotic use or changes in diet.

Role in Disease and Health:

Imbalances in the gut microbiome, known as dysbiosis, have been associated with various health conditions, including inflammatory bowel diseases (IBD), irritable bowel syndrome (IBS), obesity, and even neurological disorders.

Understanding the complexities of the gut microbiome is a rapidly evolving field of research. The significance of maintaining a healthy and diverse gut microbiome has led to lifestyle and dietary interventions aimed at promoting its well-being, reflecting the central role this microbial community plays in human health.

CONNECTION BETWEEN GUT HEALTH AND OVERALL WELL-BEING

The connection between gut health and overall well-being is a profound and intricate relationship that extends well beyond the realm of digestion. Research has unveiled a complex interplay between the gut and various aspects of physical, mental, and even emotional health. Here are key dimensions that highlight the connection between gut health and overall well-being:

• Nutrient Absorption and Energy Balance:

A healthy gut is crucial for the efficient absorption of nutrients from the food we consume. Nutrients play a vital role in energy production, cellular function, and overall metabolic balance, influencing our energy levels and general vitality.

• Immune System Regulation:

The gut is a hub for immune system activity, and a well-balanced gut microbiome is essential for a properly functioning immune response. A healthy immune system is vital for defending the body against infections and diseases, contributing to overall physical well-being.

• Inflammation and Chronic Diseases:

Chronic inflammation, often linked to imbalances in the gut microbiome, is a common factor in various chronic diseases, including cardiovascular disease, diabetes, and autoimmune conditions. A healthy gut can help regulate inflammation and mitigate the risk of these diseases.

• Gut-Brain Axis and Mental Health:

The gut and the brain communicate bidirectionally through the gut-brain axis. The state of the gut microbiome can influence mental health, mood, and cognitive function. Imbalances in the gut have been associated with conditions such as anxiety, depression, and stress.

- Gastrointestinal Health:

Of course, a primary aspect of the connection between gut health and overall well-being is the direct impact on gastrointestinal health. A well-functioning gut helps prevent digestive issues such as bloating, constipation, and diarrhea, contributing to overall comfort and quality of life.

- Neurological Conditions:

Emerging research suggests that imbalances in the gut microbiome may be linked to neurological conditions such as Parkinson's and Alzheimer's diseases. The intricate connection between the gut and the central nervous system underscores the far-reaching effects of gut health.

- Hormonal Balance:

The gut microbiome can influence hormonal balance, including hormones related to metabolism and appetite regulation. This connection is significant in the context of weight management and overall hormonal health.

• Detoxification and Waste Elimination:

A healthy gut aids in the efficient elimination of waste and toxins from the body. Proper detoxification processes contribute to overall systemic health and prevent the build-up of harmful substances.

• Impact on Sleep:

Recent studies suggest a potential link between gut health and sleep quality. Disruptions in the gut microbiome have been associated with sleep disorders, highlighting another layer of the connection between gut health and overall well-being.

Recognizing and nurturing the connection between gut health and overall well-being has given rise to the Gut Health Revolution, emphasizing lifestyle and dietary interventions aimed at promoting a balanced and thriving gut microbiome. Prioritizing gut health is increasingly viewed as a cornerstone of holistic well-being, fostering a comprehensive approach to health that encompasses both the physical and mental dimensions of our lives.

The gut microbiome is a diverse and dynamic community of microorganisms that inhabit the gastrointestinal tract, influencing various aspects of human health. This complex ecosystem is predominantly composed of bacteria, but it also includes viruses, fungi, archaea, and other microbes. Here's an overview of the major components of the gut microbiome:

1. Bacteria:

• Bacteroidetes: This phylum of bacteria is abundant in the human gut and is associated with the digestion of complex carbohydrates and the production of short-chain fatty acids (SCFAs), which have various health benefits.

• Firmicutes: Another major phylum, Firmicutes, plays a role in breaking down dietary fiber and producing energy. Imbalances in the ratio of Bacteroidetes to Firmicutes have been linked to conditions like obesity.

2. Viruses (Bacteriophages):

Bacteriophages are viruses that infect and replicate within bacteria. They are a crucial component of the gut microbiome, participating in the regulation of bacterial populations and influencing microbial diversity.

3. Fungi:

Although less studied than bacteria, fungi form a part of the gut microbiome. The most prevalent fungal species in the gut include Saccharomyces and Candida. Maintaining a balance between beneficial and harmful fungi is essential for gut health.

4. Archaea:

Archaea are single-celled microorganisms that thrive in diverse environments, including the human gut. Methanogens, a type of archaea, play a role in the metabolism of certain compounds and contribute to the overall balance of the gut ecosystem.

5. Protozoa:

Protozoa are single-celled eukaryotic organisms found in the gut. While they are not as numerous as bacteria, they contribute to the diversity of the microbiome and can interact with other microbial inhabitants.

6. Other Microbes:

Various other microorganisms, including viruses and small eukaryotes, contribute to the overall diversity of the gut microbiome. Understanding the roles and interactions of these less-studied components is an active area of research.

It's essential to note that the composition of the gut microbiome is highly individualized, influenced by factors such as genetics, diet, age, and environmental exposures. Moreover, the balance of these microbial components is crucial for maintaining a healthy gut. Imbalances, known as dysbiosis, can lead to various health issues and are associated with conditions such as inflammatory bowel diseases (IBD), irritable bowel syndrome (IBS), and metabolic disorders.

The diversity and complexity of the gut microbiome highlight its importance in supporting digestion, immune function, and overall well-being. Ongoing research is continuously uncovering the intricate relationships between the various components of the gut microbiome and their impact on human health.

The gut microbiome plays a crucial role in digestion, contributing to the breakdown of complex dietary components and influencing the absorption of nutrients. This intricate relationship between the gut microbiome and digestion has far-reaching effects on overall health. Here's an exploration of the key roles the gut microbiome plays in the digestive process:

1. Fermentation of Dietary Fiber:

The gut microbiome excels at breaking down complex carbohydrates, particularly dietary fiber that escapes digestion in the small intestine. Bacterial fermentation of fiber produces short-chain fatty acids (SCFAs), such as acetate, propionate, and butyrate. SCFAs serve as an energy source for the cells lining the colon and contribute to overall gut health.

2. Production of Enzymes:

Some bacteria in the gut microbiome produce enzymes that aid in the digestion of specific compounds. For example, certain bacteria help break down complex sugars and starches that the human digestive enzymes may not fully process in the upper gastrointestinal tract.

3. Metabolism of Undigested Carbohydrates:

The gut microbiome assists in the metabolism of carbohydrates that escape digestion in the small intestine. Bacteria can convert these undigested carbohydrates into various byproducts, including gases like hydrogen and methane.

4. Amino Acid Metabolism:

Certain bacteria in the gut contribute to the breakdown of proteins into amino acids. This process not only aids in the absorption of essential amino acids but also generates byproducts that may have implications for overall health.

5. Bile Acid Metabolism:

The gut microbiome plays a role in the metabolism of bile acids, which are essential for the digestion and absorption of fats. Bacteria in the colon can modify bile acids, influencing their composition and signaling properties.

6. Vitamin Synthesis:

Some bacteria in the gut microbiome contribute to the synthesis of certain vitamins, including B vitamins (such as B12, biotin, and folate) and vitamin K. These vitamins are crucial for various physiological processes, including blood clotting and energy metabolism.

7. Detoxification of Xenobiotics:

The gut microbiome has the ability to metabolize and detoxify certain compounds, including drugs and environmental toxins. This detoxification process helps protect the host from harmful substances.

8. Maintenance of Gut Barrier Function:

The gut microbiome contributes to the maintenance of the intestinal barrier, preventing the entry of harmful substances into the bloodstream. A healthy gut barrier is essential for overall digestive health and immune function.

9. Regulation of Gastrointestinal Motility:

The gut microbiome can influence the movement of the gastrointestinal tract, regulating gut motility. This can impact the rate at which food moves through the digestive system, influencing nutrient absorption and stool formation.

Understanding the integral role of the gut microbiome in digestion highlights its significance in maintaining not only digestive health but also overall well-being. Imbalances in the gut microbiome can lead to dysregulation of these processes, contributing to digestive disorders and other health issues. As a result, promoting a healthy gut microbiome through a balanced diet, prebiotics, and probiotics is crucial for optimal digestion and overall health.

GUT-IMMUNE SYSTEM INTERACTION

The interaction between the gut and the immune system is a dynamic and intricate relationship that plays a central role in maintaining overall health. The gut is a major interface between the external environment (including the diverse array of microorganisms in the digestive tract) and the internal milieu of the body. The gut-associated lymphoid tissue (GALT) and the gut microbiome are key components in this interaction. Here's an exploration of the gut-immune system connection:

1. Gut-Associated Lymphoid Tissue (GALT):

The GALT is a specialized component of the immune system located in the lining of the gastrointestinal tract. It includes lymphoid follicles, Peyer's patches, and other immune cells strategically positioned to monitor and respond to potential threats from the gut environment.

2. Immunoglobulin Production:

The gut-associated lymphoid tissue is involved in the production of immunoglobulins, including IgA. Immunoglobulin A (IgA) is a crucial antibody that plays a primary role in mucosal immunity, providing a defense mechanism against pathogens in the gut lumen.

3. Tolerance and Regulation:

The gut immune system is tasked with distinguishing between harmful pathogens and beneficial microbes to maintain a state of immune tolerance. This delicate balance allows the immune system to respond appropriately to threats while avoiding unnecessary inflammation in response to harmless antigens.

4. Microbial Recognition:

Immune cells in the gut are equipped with pattern recognition receptors (PRRs) that can identify specific molecular patterns associated with microorganisms. This recognition helps the immune system differentiate between beneficial and harmful microbes.

5. Inflammatory Responses:

When pathogens breach the mucosal barrier or when there's an imbalance in the gut microbiome, the immune system may initiate controlled inflammatory responses. Inflammation is a crucial defense mechanism but must be tightly regulated to prevent chronic inflammation and associated health issues.

6. T-Cell Regulation:

Specialized T cells, including regulatory T cells (Tregs), play a critical role in regulating immune responses in the gut. Tregs help maintain immune tolerance, preventing excessive inflammation and autoimmune reactions.

7. Communication via Cytokines:

Immune cells in the gut communicate with each other and with the gut microbiome through the release of signaling molecules called cytokines. Cytokines coordinate immune responses and help modulate the activity of immune cells.

8. Impact on Systemic Immunity:

The gut immune system has systemic effects, influencing immune responses throughout the body. Disruptions in gut health have been linked to various systemic conditions, emphasizing the importance of a healthy gut for overall immune function.

9. Role in Autoimmune Diseases:

Dysregulation in the gut-immune system interaction has been implicated in the development of autoimmune diseases. Imbalances in the gut microbiome and compromised gut barrier function may contribute to the initiation or exacerbation of autoimmune conditions.

Understanding the crosstalk between the gut and the immune system is essential for appreciating the broader implications of gut health on overall well-being. A balanced and diverse gut microbiome, along with a well-regulated immune response, is crucial for maintaining immune homeostasis and preventing conditions associated with immune dysfunction. Strategies to support gut health, including a healthy diet, probiotics, and lifestyle modifications, can positively impact this intricate relationship.

DEFENSE AGAINST PATHOGENS

The gut plays a critical role in defending the body against pathogens, harmful microorganisms that can cause infections and diseases. The defense mechanisms in the gut involve a complex interplay between the gut-associated lymphoid tissue (GALT), the gut microbiome, and various components of the immune system. Here's an exploration of how the gut serves as a frontline defender against pathogens:

1. Gut-Associated Lymphoid Tissue (GALT):

The GALT is a network of specialized immune tissues and cells lining the gastrointestinal tract. It includes lymph nodes,

Peyer's patches, and immune cells strategically positioned to detect and respond to pathogens entering the gut.

2. Immunoglobulin Production:

The GALT is involved in the production of immunoglobulins, particularly Immunoglobulin A (IgA). IgA is a primary antibody that plays a crucial role in mucosal immunity. It helps neutralize and eliminate pathogens in the gut lumen, preventing them from entering the bloodstream.

3. Mucosal Barrier Function:

The mucosal lining of the gut acts as a physical barrier that prevents pathogens from directly accessing the underlying tissues. Tight junctions between epithelial cells form a protective barrier, and mucins, secreted by goblet cells, create a barrier that traps and expels pathogens.

4. Microbial Competition and Exclusion:

The presence of a diverse and healthy gut microbiome creates a competitive environment for pathogens. Beneficial microbes can outcompete pathogens for nutrients and adhesion sites, limiting the ability of harmful organisms to establish infections.

5. Antimicrobial Peptides:

The gut produces various antimicrobial peptides, small proteins with the ability to kill or inhibit the growth of pathogens. These peptides contribute to the defense against a wide range of microorganisms.

6. Phagocytosis by Immune Cells:

Immune cells, such as macrophages and dendritic cells, patrol the gut mucosa, identifying and engulfing pathogens. This process, known as phagocytosis, helps neutralize and eliminate potential threats.

7. T-Cell Responses:

T cells, including cytotoxic T cells, play a role in recognizing and eliminating infected cells. Regulatory T cells help modulate immune responses, preventing excessive inflammation while maintaining effective defense against pathogens.

8. Inflammatory Responses:

In response to the presence of pathogens, the immune system may initiate controlled inflammatory responses. Inflammation is a protective mechanism aimed at eliminating the threat, but it needs to be regulated to avoid excessive tissue damage.

9. Adaptive Immune Memory:

Following exposure to pathogens, the immune system develops memory cells that "remember" the encountered pathogens. This adaptive immune memory allows for a faster and more robust response upon subsequent exposures, providing long-lasting protection.

10. Cytokine Signaling:

Cytokines are signaling molecules released by immune cells to coordinate and regulate immune responses. In the context of defending against pathogens, cytokines play a crucial role in communication between immune cells and in the recruitment of additional immune cells to the site of infection.

Understanding the multifaceted defense mechanisms in the gut highlights its significance in protecting the body from infections. Maintaining a healthy gut microbiome, supporting mucosal barrier function, and promoting a well-regulated immune response are essential for effective defense against pathogens and overall immune health.

CHAPTER TWO

IMPORTANCE OF FIBER

Dietary fiber is a crucial component of a healthy diet, offering a range of benefits that contribute to overall well-being. It is found in plant-based foods and comes in two main forms: soluble fiber, which dissolves in water, and insoluble fiber, which does not dissolve. Here are key reasons highlighting the importance of including an adequate amount of fiber in your diet:

Digestive Health:

• Preventing Constipation: Insoluble fiber adds bulk to the stool and helps prevent constipation by promoting regular bowel movements.

• Maintaining Bowel Regularity: Both soluble and insoluble fiber contribute to maintaining optimal bowel regularity, preventing diarrhea or constipation.

Weight Management:

• Enhancing Satiety: High-fiber foods are often more filling, promoting a feeling of fullness. This can help with weight management by reducing overall calorie intake.

Blood Sugar Control:

• Stabilizing Blood Glucose Levels: Soluble fiber, particularly found in foods like oats and legumes, can help stabilize blood sugar levels by slowing down the absorption of sugar.

Heart Health:

• Lowering Cholesterol Levels: Soluble fiber can help lower LDL (bad) cholesterol levels by binding to cholesterol particles and aiding in their excretion.

• Reducing Blood Pressure: Some studies suggest that a high-fiber diet may contribute to lower blood pressure levels, reducing the risk of cardiovascular diseases.

Management of Type 2 Diabetes:

• Improving Insulin Sensitivity: Soluble fiber can contribute to improved insulin sensitivity, which is beneficial for individuals with type 2 diabetes.

Gut Microbiome Health:

• Promoting a Diverse Microbiome: Fiber serves as a source of nutrition for beneficial gut bacteria, promoting the growth of a diverse and healthy gut microbiome.

• Fermentation and Short-Chain Fatty Acids: Some types of fiber are fermented by gut bacteria, leading to the production of short-chain fatty acids (SCFAs), which have various health benefits.

Prevention of Colorectal Cancer:

• Reducing Cancer Risk: High-fiber diets, particularly those rich in insoluble fiber, are associated with a lower risk of colorectal cancer.

Immune Function:

• Supporting Immune Response: A healthy gut microbiome, influenced by fiber intake, plays a crucial role in supporting immune function and defending against infections.

Inflammation Reduction:

• Anti-Inflammatory Effects: Soluble fiber may contribute to reducing inflammation in the body, which is linked to various chronic diseases.

Supporting Healthy Aging:

• Cognitive Health: Some studies suggest that a diet rich in fiber may contribute to cognitive health and a lower risk of age-related cognitive decline.

Disease Prevention:

• Reducing Risk of Chronic Diseases: Adequate fiber intake is associated with a lower risk of developing various chronic diseases, including heart disease, diabetes, and certain types of cancer.

It's important to note that obtaining fiber from a variety of sources, including fruits, vegetables, whole grains, legumes, and nuts, is ideal for reaping the full spectrum of benefits. The recommended daily intake of fiber varies by age, sex, and other factors, but in general, most health organizations suggest aiming for at least 25 grams of fiber per day for adults. Including a diverse range of fiber-rich foods in your diet is a simple yet impactful way to support your overall health and well-being.

PROBIOTICS AND PREBIOTICS

Probiotics and prebiotics are terms often associated with gut health, and they play distinct but complementary roles in supporting the well-being of the gastrointestinal system. Let's explore the definitions and roles of both probiotics and prebiotics:

Probiotics:

Definition: Probiotics are live microorganisms, mainly bacteria and yeast, that confer health benefits to the host when consumed in adequate amounts. They are often referred to as "good" or "friendly" bacteria and contribute to the balance of the gut microbiome.

Roles and Benefits:

• Maintaining Gut Microbiome Balance: Probiotics help balance the composition of the gut microbiome by promoting the growth of beneficial bacteria.

• Digestive Health: They assist in the breakdown of food, enhance nutrient absorption, and contribute to overall digestive health.

• Immune System Support: Probiotics play a role in supporting the immune system and can help regulate immune responses.

• Prevention of Diarrhea: Certain strains of probiotics have been shown to be effective in preventing or alleviating diarrhea, especially antibiotic-associated diarrhea.

• Management of Irritable Bowel Syndrome (IBS): Probiotics may provide relief for some symptoms associated with IBS, such as abdominal pain and bloating.

• Potential Mental Health Benefits: Emerging research suggests a link between gut health, probiotics, and mental well-being, with some studies indicating a positive impact on mood and anxiety.

• Sources: Probiotics can be found in various fermented foods and dietary supplements. Common sources include yogurt, kefir, sauerkraut, kimchi, miso, and certain types of pickles.

Prebiotics:

Definition: Prebiotics are non-digestible fibers and compounds that serve as a food source for beneficial bacteria in the gut. Unlike probiotics, prebiotics are not living organisms but rather substances that promote the growth and activity of existing beneficial bacteria.

Roles and Benefits:

• Nourishing Beneficial Bacteria: Prebiotics provide a substrate for the growth and activity of beneficial bacteria, particularly those that contribute to a healthy gut microbiome.

• Colon Health: They help maintain the health of the colon by supporting the growth of mucosal cells and promoting the production of short-chain fatty acids (SCFAs).

• Regulating Blood Sugar Levels: Prebiotics may contribute to improved insulin sensitivity, helping to regulate blood sugar levels.

• Supporting Calcium Absorption: Some prebiotics, such as inulin, have been associated with improved calcium absorption, benefiting bone health.

• Enhancing Mineral Absorption: Prebiotics may facilitate the absorption of other minerals, such as magnesium and iron.

• Potential Weight Management: There is some evidence suggesting that prebiotics may contribute to weight management by promoting satiety and influencing energy balance.

• Sources: Prebiotics are naturally present in various plant-based foods. Common sources include chicory root, garlic, onions, leeks, bananas, asparagus, Jerusalem artichokes, and whole grains.

Synbiotics:

Definition: Synbiotics refer to products that combine both probiotics and prebiotics, aiming to enhance the survival and activity of the beneficial microorganisms in the gut.

Roles and Benefits:

• Optimizing Gut Health: Synbiotics work synergistically to support the growth and activity of beneficial bacteria in the gut, promoting overall gut health.

• Improved Viability: Prebiotics serve as a source of nourishment for probiotics, enhancing their viability and effectiveness.

Probiotics and prebiotics, whether consumed separately or together as synbiotics, contribute to the maintenance of a healthy gut microbiome, supporting various aspects of digestion, immune function, and overall well-being. Including a variety of probiotic-rich and prebiotic-containing foods in the diet can be a valuable strategy for promoting gut health. Additionally, if considering supplements, it's advisable to consult with a healthcare professional for personalized recommendations.

INFLUENCE OF EXERCISE ON GUT HEALTH

Exercise has a notable influence on gut health, contributing to the overall well-being of the gastrointestinal system and the gut microbiome. The connection between physical activity and gut health is a dynamic and multifaceted relationship, and research suggests several positive effects. Here are key ways in which exercise influences gut health:

Diversity of Gut Microbiome:

• Increased Microbial Diversity: Regular exercise has been associated with an increase in the diversity of the gut microbiome. A more diverse microbiome is often considered a marker of good gut health.

Anti-Inflammatory Effects:

• Reduced Inflammation: Exercise has anti-inflammatory effects, and chronic inflammation in the gut is linked to various gastrointestinal conditions. Regular physical activity may contribute to a more balanced inflammatory response.

Metabolic Health:

• Improved Insulin Sensitivity: Exercise improves insulin sensitivity, and this positive impact on metabolic health may indirectly influence the gut microbiome and reduce the risk of metabolic disorders.

Promotion of Butyrate Production:

• Increased Short-Chain Fatty Acids (SCFAs): Exercise has been associated with higher levels of short-chain fatty acids (SCFAs), including butyrate. SCFAs play a role in maintaining gut health and have various benefits for the host.

Gut Motility:

• Enhanced Gut Motility: Regular physical activity can help regulate bowel movements and enhance gut motility. This may contribute to the prevention of constipation and other digestive issues.

Stress Reduction:

• Reduced Stress Levels: Exercise is known to reduce stress, and stress management is crucial for gut health. Chronic stress has been linked to gut disorders, and exercise can mitigate stress-related impacts on the gastrointestinal system.

Immune Function:

• Enhanced Immune Response: Regular moderate exercise has been associated with improvements in immune function. A robust immune system is essential for protecting the gut from infections and maintaining overall health.

Brain-Gut Axis Interaction:

• Influence on the Gut-Brain Axis: Exercise may impact the gut-brain axis, the bidirectional communication between the gut and the central nervous system. This connection can influence mood, mental well-being, and aspects of gastrointestinal function.

Weight Management:

• Contribution to Weight Management: Regular physical activity plays a role in weight management, and maintaining a healthy weight is associated with better gut health.

Epigenetic Changes:

• Epigenetic Modifications: Exercise can induce epigenetic changes, influencing gene expression in cells, including those in the gut. These changes may have positive effects on various physiological processes.

Improved Circulation:

• Enhanced Blood Flow: Exercise promotes better blood circulation, which can contribute to improved nutrient delivery to the gut and support the overall health of the gastrointestinal tissues.

It's important to note that individual responses to exercise can vary, and excessive or intense exercise may have different effects on gut health than moderate, regular physical activity.

As with any health-related consideration, it's advisable to consult with healthcare professionals, including a healthcare provider or a registered dietitian, for personalized advice on incorporating exercise into one's routine to promote gut health.

INFLUENCE OF SLEEP ON GUT HEALTH

The relationship between sleep and gut health is bidirectional, with each influencing the other. A lack of quality sleep or irregular sleep patterns can negatively impact the gut, and conversely, a healthy gut can contribute to better sleep. Here are key aspects of the influence of sleep on gut health:

1. Gut Motility and Digestion:

• Sleep and Gut Motility: Sleep is associated with changes in gut motility, and disruptions to sleep patterns can influence the rhythmic contractions of the digestive tract. Irregular gut motility may contribute to digestive issues.

2. Gut Microbiome:

• Impact on Microbial Composition: Sleep disturbances, such as insufficient or poor-quality sleep, have been linked to alterations in the composition and diversity of the gut microbiome. Changes in the microbiome may affect overall gut health.

3. Inflammation:

• Influence on Inflammatory Responses: Lack of sleep has been associated with increased levels of systemic inflammation. Chronic inflammation can impact the gut, potentially leading to conditions like inflammatory bowel disease (IBD) or irritable bowel syndrome (IBS).

4. Intestinal Barrier Function:

• Disruption of Barrier Integrity: Poor sleep quality may compromise the integrity of the intestinal barrier. A weakened barrier can lead to increased permeability, allowing substances to enter the bloodstream and potentially triggering inflammatory responses.

5. Hormonal Regulation:

• Effects on Hormones: Sleep influences the release of hormones, including those that regulate appetite and metabolism. Disruptions to these hormonal signals may contribute to weight gain and metabolic imbalances, affecting gut health.

6. Immune Function:

• Reduced Immune Function: Inadequate sleep has been associated with a weakened immune system. A compromised immune response can make the gut more susceptible to infections and inflammation.

7. Circadian Rhythms:

• Synchronization with Circadian Rhythms: The gut microbiome follows a circadian rhythm, influenced by the body's internal clock. Irregular sleep patterns or disruptions to circadian rhythms may impact the timing and effectiveness of certain gut processes.

8. Gut-Brain Axis:

• Communication with the Brain: The gut and the brain communicate through the gut-brain axis. Sleep disturbances may affect this communication, potentially influencing mood, stress levels, and cognitive function.

9. Impact on Gut Disorders:

• Association with Gastrointestinal Disorders: Sleep disturbances have been linked to an increased risk of developing certain gastrointestinal disorders, including functional gastrointestinal disorders like IBS.

10. Food Choices:

• Influence on Dietary Patterns: Poor sleep has been associated with altered food choices, including a preference for high-calorie, sugary foods. Dietary habits can impact the gut microbiome and overall gut health.

11. Stress Levels:

• Increased Stress Levels: Sleep deprivation can increase stress levels, and chronic stress is associated with gut issues such as irritable bowel syndrome (IBS) and inflammatory bowel disease (IBD).

12. Quality of Life:

• Overall Well-Being: Adequate sleep is crucial for overall well-being, and a lack of quality sleep may contribute to stress, anxiety, and a reduced quality of life, all of which can affect gut health.

Maintaining a regular sleep schedule, prioritizing sufficient sleep, and practicing good sleep hygiene are essential for promoting both overall health and gut health. Conversely, a healthy gut, achieved through a balanced diet, regular physical activity, and gut-friendly habits, can contribute to better sleep patterns and overall well-being. If sleep disturbances persist or if gut issues are a concern, it's advisable to consult with healthcare professionals for personalized guidance and intervention.

INFLUENCE OF STRESS ON GUT HEALTH

Stress can have a significant impact on gut health, and the connection between the two is often referred to as the "gut-brain axis." The gut-brain axis represents the bidirectional communication between the central nervous system (including the brain) and the enteric nervous system of the gut. Stress can influence various aspects of gastrointestinal function and is associated with the development or exacerbation of certain gastrointestinal disorders. Here are key ways in which stress affects gut health:

1. Changes in Gut Motility:

• Increased or Decreased Motility: Stress can lead to alterations in gut motility, resulting in either increased or decreased movement of the digestive tract. This can contribute to symptoms such as diarrhea or constipation.

2. Altered Intestinal Permeability:

• Leaky Gut Syndrome: Chronic stress may contribute to increased intestinal permeability, commonly referred to as "leaky gut." This allows substances that are normally restricted to the digestive tract to pass into the bloodstream, potentially triggering inflammatory responses.

3. Inflammation:

• Immune System Activation: Stress activates the immune system, leading to the release of inflammatory molecules. Chronic inflammation in the gut is associated with conditions like inflammatory bowel disease (IBD) and irritable bowel syndrome (IBS).

4. Changes in Gut Microbiome:

• Microbial Imbalances: Stress can influence the composition and diversity of the gut microbiome. Imbalances in the microbial community may contribute to gastrointestinal symptoms and impact overall gut health.

5. Visceral Hypersensitivity:

• Increased Sensitivity: Stress may heighten the perception of pain in the gut, leading to visceral hypersensitivity. Individuals experiencing stress may be more prone to feeling discomfort or pain in response to normal gut stimuli.

6. Gastrointestinal Disorders:

• Exacerbation of Symptoms: Stress is known to exacerbate symptoms in individuals with existing gastrointestinal disorders such as irritable bowel syndrome (IBS), inflammatory bowel disease (IBD), and functional dyspepsia.

7. Alterations in Gut Hormones:

• Hormonal Changes: Stress can influence the release of gut hormones, affecting digestive processes and appetite regulation. Dysregulation of these hormones may contribute to gastrointestinal symptoms.

8. Impact on Gut-Brain Axis:

• Communication Disruptions: Chronic stress may disrupt the communication between the gut and the brain through the gut-brain axis, influencing mood, cognitive function, and emotional well-being.

9. Effects on Mucosal Barrier Function:

• Compromised Barrier Function: Stress may compromise the integrity of the mucosal barrier in the gut, leading to increased permeability. This can allow harmful substances to enter the bloodstream, potentially contributing to inflammation.

10. Modulation of Immune Responses:

• Altered Immune Function: Chronic stress can modulate immune responses in the gut, potentially contributing to an increased susceptibility to infections or the development of autoimmune conditions.

11. Functional Gastrointestinal Disorders:

• Triggers for Symptoms: Stress is often recognized as a trigger for symptoms in functional gastrointestinal disorders like IBS, where symptoms may be exacerbated during times of stress.

12. Potential Contribution to Gastrointestinal Diseases:

• Association with Disease Onset: While stress alone may not cause gastrointestinal diseases, it is thought to play a role in disease onset and exacerbation, particularly in genetically predisposed individuals.

13. Impacts on Dietary Habits:

• Changes in Eating Patterns: Stress may influence dietary habits, leading to changes in food choices. This, in turn, can impact the gut microbiome and digestive processes.

14. Connection to Mental Health:

• Bidirectional Influence: The gut-brain axis reflects the bidirectional communication between the gut and the brain. Stress-related changes in the gut can, in turn, influence mental health and emotional well-being.

Managing stress through techniques such as relaxation, mindfulness, and stress-reduction strategies may positively impact gut health. Additionally, maintaining a healthy lifestyle, including a balanced diet and regular physical activity, can contribute to overall well-being and support the health of the gut-brain axis. Individuals experiencing persistent gastrointestinal symptoms or stress-related health concerns should consult with healthcare professionals for proper evaluation and guidance.

INFLUENCE OF ANTIBIOTIC USE ON GUT HEALTH

Antibiotics are medications designed to kill or inhibit the growth of bacteria, and while they are essential for treating bacterial infections, their use can have significant implications for gut health. Antibiotics are not selective in their action, meaning they can affect both harmful and beneficial bacteria in the gut. Here are key ways in which antibiotic use can influence gut health:

• Alteration in Microbial Composition: Antibiotics can lead to a significant disruption in the balance and diversity of the gut microbiome. They may reduce the abundance of beneficial bacteria, allowing opportunistic or harmful bacteria to thrive.

• Reduced Microbial Diversity: Antibiotic use is associated with a decrease in microbial diversity in the gut. A less diverse microbiome is often linked to various health issues.

• Proliferation of Harmful Bacteria: The depletion of beneficial bacteria can create an environment in which opportunistic pathogens, such as Clostridium difficile, can overgrow and cause infections, leading to conditions like antibiotic-associated diarrhea or pseudomembranous colitis.

• Reduced Short-Chain Fatty Acids (SCFAs): Antibiotic-induced changes in the gut microbiome can lead to a decrease in the production of short-chain fatty acids (SCFAs), which play a crucial role in gut health and immune function.

• Changes in Nutrient Metabolism: Antibiotics can affect the metabolism of dietary compounds, influencing the breakdown and absorption of nutrients. This may have implications for overall nutritional status.

• Weakened Intestinal Barrier: Disruption of the gut microbiome by antibiotics can compromise the integrity of the intestinal barrier. A weakened barrier may lead to increased permeability, allowing substances to enter the bloodstream and triggering inflammatory responses.

• Increased Risk of Gastrointestinal Issues: Long-term or repeated antibiotic use has been associated with an increased risk of developing gastrointestinal issues, including irritable bowel syndrome (IBS) and inflammatory bowel disease (IBD).

• Increased Vulnerability to Infections: While antibiotics are used to treat infections, their use can also make individuals more susceptible to new infections due to the disruption of the normal protective microbiota.

• Development of Antibiotic Resistance: The use of antibiotics can contribute to the development of antibiotic-resistant strains of bacteria. This is a global health concern that can impact the effectiveness of antibiotic treatments in the future.

• Potential Impact on Metabolic Health: Some studies suggest that early antibiotic exposure, especially in infancy, may have long-term effects on metabolism, potentially influencing weight and metabolic health.

• Modulation of Immune Responses: Antibiotic-induced changes in the gut microbiome can influence immune system function. Altered immune responses may contribute to increased susceptibility to certain diseases or autoimmune conditions.

• Influence of Timing and Duration: The timing and duration of antibiotic use can affect the extent of disruption to the gut microbiome. Short-term use may have less profound effects compared to prolonged or frequent use.

• Differences in Individual Responses: Individuals may respond differently to antibiotic treatment, with some experiencing more pronounced disruptions to the gut microbiome than others. Factors such as genetics, diet, and overall health can contribute to this variability.

• Gradual Restoration: After completing a course of antibiotics, the gut microbiome can gradually recover. However, the extent of recovery and the composition of the microbiome may vary among individuals.

• Role of Probiotics: Some individuals may use probiotics, which are beneficial bacteria, during or after antibiotic treatment to help restore the balance of the gut microbiome. However, the efficacy of probiotics in this context is still an active area of research.

• Proactive Measures: In certain situations, healthcare providers may take preventive measures, such as prescribing probiotics alongside antibiotics or recommending strategies to support gut health during and after antibiotic use.

It's important to note that while antibiotics are essential for treating bacterial infections, their use should be judicious, and healthcare providers carefully consider the potential impacts on gut health. When prescribed antibiotics, individuals are encouraged to follow their healthcare provider's instructions, complete the full course of treatment, and communicate any concerns or side effects. Additionally, focusing on strategies to support gut health, such as a balanced diet and the use of probiotics, may be considered in consultation with healthcare professionals.

CHAPTER THREE

An unhealthy gut can manifest in various signs and symptoms, indicating an imbalance in the gut microbiome, compromised gut barrier function, or other gastrointestinal issues. Here are some common signs of an unhealthy gut:

1. Digestive Issues:

• Chronic Constipation or Diarrhea: Persistent constipation or diarrhea can be signs of gastrointestinal distress.

• Gas and Bloating: Excessive gas production and abdominal bloating after meals may indicate gut issues.

2. Food Intolerances or Sensitivities:

• Reactions to Certain Foods: Intolerance or sensitivity to certain foods, such as gluten or dairy, may suggest gut health issues.

3. Chronic Fatigue or Low Energy Levels:

• Persistent Fatigue: Ongoing fatigue or low energy levels despite adequate rest may be linked to poor gut health.

4. Mood Changes:

• Anxiety or Depression: Mood disorders like anxiety or depression may be associated with alterations in the gut-brain axis.

5. Skin Conditions:

• Acne, Eczema, or Psoriasis: Skin conditions may be exacerbated by imbalances in the gut microbiome.

6. Unintentional Weight Changes:

• Unexplained Weight Gain or Loss: Significant changes in weight without changes in diet or exercise habits may signal gut issues.

7. Autoimmune Conditions:

• Development or Exacerbation of Autoimmune Diseases: Certain autoimmune conditions, such as rheumatoid arthritis or inflammatory bowel disease, may be linked to gut health.

8. Sugar Cravings:

• Cravings for Sugary Foods: Intense cravings for sugary foods may indicate dysbiosis in the gut microbiome.

9. Recurrent Infections:

• Frequent Infections: Increased susceptibility to infections may suggest an impaired immune system, possibly related to gut health.

10. Joint Pain:

• Joint Pain or Inflammation: Inflammation in the gut can sometimes manifest as joint pain or inflammation.

11. Sleep Disturbances:

• Difficulty Sleeping: Insomnia or disrupted sleep patterns may be linked to gut health issues, given the influence of the gut microbiome on sleep regulation.

12. Brain Fog or Cognitive Issues:

• Difficulty Concentrating: Cognitive issues such as brain fog or difficulty concentrating may be associated with gut-brain axis dysfunction.

13. Chronic Bad Breath:

• Persistent Halitosis: Chronic bad breath that does not improve with oral hygiene measures may be related to gut issues.

14. Chronic Stress:

• Heightened Stress Levels: Chronic stress can negatively impact gut health and may exacerbate existing gastrointestinal symptoms.

15. Nutritional Deficiencies:

• Deficiencies in Essential Nutrients: Malabsorption or poor nutrient absorption due to gut issues can lead to deficiencies in vitamins and minerals.

16. Frequent Headaches:

• Regular Headaches or Migraines: Gut dysbiosis and inflammation may contribute to headaches or migraines in some individuals.

17. Autoimmune Skin Conditions:

• Psoriasis or Eczema: Some autoimmune skin conditions may be linked to gut health, as inflammation in the gut can affect systemic inflammation.

18. Increased Sensitivity to Medications:

• Heightened Sensitivity to Medications: Individuals with gut issues may experience increased sensitivity to certain medications or side effects.

19. Frequent Antibiotic Use:

• Recurring Antibiotic Use: Frequent use of antibiotics can disrupt the gut microbiome, leading to gut health issues.

20. Poor Oral Health:

• Gum Disease or Tooth Decay: Poor oral health, including gum disease or tooth decay, may be associated with imbalances in the gut microbiome.

If you experience several of these symptoms persistently, it may be advisable to consult with a healthcare professional, such as a gastroenterologist or a registered dietitian, for proper evaluation and guidance. Addressing underlying gut health issues may involve dietary modifications, lifestyle changes, probiotic supplementation, and other targeted interventions tailored to individual needs.

SKIN CONDITIONS AS A RESULT OF UNHEALTHY GUT

The gut-skin connection is a growing area of research, and emerging evidence suggests that the health of the gut microbiome can influence various aspects of skin health. An unhealthy gut, characterized by imbalances in the gut microbiota, inflammation, and compromised gut barrier function, may contribute to or exacerbate certain skin conditions. While more research is needed to fully understand the complex interactions between the gut and skin, here are some skin conditions that may be influenced by an unhealthy gut:

• Acne: Imbalances in the gut microbiome and increased intestinal permeability (leaky gut) may contribute to systemic inflammation, influencing acne development.

• Eczema (Dermatitis): Alterations in gut microbiota composition, immune system dysregulation, and increased intestinal permeability may play a role in the development or exacerbation of eczema.

• Psoriasis: Imbalances in the gut microbiome and dysregulation of the immune system may contribute to the inflammatory processes associated with psoriasis.

• Rosacea: Intestinal dysbiosis and increased gut permeability may be associated with systemic inflammation, potentially influencing rosacea symptoms.

• Dermatitis Herpetiformis: Dermatitis herpetiformis is associated with celiac disease, an autoimmune condition triggered by gluten consumption. The gut-skin connection is evident in this gluten-sensitive skin condition.

• Hives (Urticaria): Gut health, particularly the balance of gut bacteria, may influence the immune system's response and contribute to the development of hives.

• Pruritus (Itchy Skin): Chronic itching without a visible rash may be associated with systemic inflammation and immune responses influenced by gut health.

• Acrodermatitis Enteropathica: This rare skin condition is associated with zinc deficiency, and malabsorption issues in the gut can contribute to zinc deficiencies.

• Skin Infections: Disruptions in gut microbiota may impact the overall immune function, potentially increasing susceptibility to skin infections.

• Atopic Dermatitis: Changes in gut microbiota composition, particularly in early life, have been associated with an increased risk of developing atopic dermatitis.

• Vitiligo: Autoimmune conditions, including those involving the skin like vitiligo, may be influenced by immune responses triggered by gut health.

• Hidradenitis Suppurativa: Inflammation and dysregulation of the immune system, both influenced by gut health, may play a role in hidradenitis suppurativa.

• Acquired Cutis Laxa: Acquired cutis laxa, characterized by loose and sagging skin, may be associated with gastrointestinal disorders that impact connective tissue.

• Cutaneous Manifestations of Gastrointestinal Disorders: Certain gastrointestinal disorders, such as Crohn's disease and ulcerative colitis, may have cutaneous manifestations, and the gut-skin connection is evident in these cases.

It's important to note that while there is growing interest in the gut-skin axis, individual responses may vary, and more research is needed to establish specific cause-and-effect relationships. Maintaining a healthy gut through a balanced diet, probiotics, and lifestyle practices may have positive effects on overall health, including skin health. If you are experiencing skin issues, it's recommended to consult with a healthcare professional or dermatologist for a comprehensive evaluation and appropriate management.

An unhealthy gut can contribute to various digestive issues, as the gut plays a central role in the digestion and absorption of nutrients. Imbalances in the gut microbiome, inflammation, and compromised gut barrier function are factors that may lead to or exacerbate digestive problems. Here are some common digestive issues that can be associated with an unhealthy gut:

1. Irritable Bowel Syndrome (IBS):

• Symptoms: Abdominal pain, bloating, gas, diarrhea, and constipation.

• Potential Link: Altered gut microbiota, intestinal inflammation, and increased gut permeability may contribute to IBS symptoms.

2. Inflammatory Bowel Disease (IBD):

• Types: Crohn's disease and ulcerative colitis.

• Symptoms: Abdominal pain, diarrhea (often bloody), weight loss, and fatigue.

• Potential Link: Chronic inflammation of the gastrointestinal tract, influenced by an immune response and gut dysbiosis.

3. Gastroesophageal Reflux Disease (GERD):

• Symptoms: Heartburn, regurgitation, chest pain, and difficulty swallowing.

• Potential Link: Disruptions in the lower esophageal sphincter and imbalances in the gut microbiome may contribute to GERD.

4. Celiac Disease:

• Symptoms: Diarrhea, abdominal pain, weight loss, and skin rashes (dermatitis herpetiformis).

• Potential Link: Autoimmune response triggered by gluten consumption, affecting the small intestine.

5. Dyspepsia (Indigestion):

• Symptoms: Upper abdominal discomfort, bloating, and early satiety.

• Potential Link: Gut dysbiosis, altered gut motility, and inflammation may contribute to indigestion.

6. Gastroenteritis:

• Symptoms: Diarrhea, nausea, vomiting, abdominal cramps, and fever.

• Potential Link: Inflammation of the gastrointestinal tract often caused by infections, affecting gut health.

7. Small Intestinal Bacterial Overgrowth (SIBO):

• Symptoms: Bloating, diarrhea, abdominal pain, and malabsorption.

• Potential Link: Abnormal overgrowth of bacteria in the small intestine, disrupting normal digestive processes.

8. Constipation:

• Symptoms: Difficulty passing stools, infrequent bowel movements, and abdominal discomfort.

• Potential Link: Imbalances in gut microbiota, inadequate fiber intake, and slowed gut motility can contribute to constipation.

9. Leaky Gut Syndrome:

• Symptoms: Abdominal pain, bloating, fatigue, joint pain, and food sensitivities.

• Potential Link: Increased intestinal permeability, allowing substances to enter the bloodstream and triggering immune responses.

10. Food Intolerances:

• Symptoms: Bloating, gas, diarrhea, and abdominal pain after consuming specific foods.

• Potential Link: Impaired digestion and altered gut permeability can lead to food intolerances.

11. Gallstones:

• Symptoms: Abdominal pain (especially after eating fatty foods), nausea, and vomiting.

• Potential Link: Imbalances in bile composition or reduced gallbladder function may contribute to gallstone formation.

12. Diverticulitis:

• Symptoms: Abdominal pain (usually on the left side), fever, nausea, and changes in bowel habits.

• Potential Link: Inflammation or infection of small pouches (diverticula) in the colon.

13. Colorectal Polyps:

• Symptoms: Often asymptomatic, but may cause bleeding, changes in bowel habits, or abdominal pain.

• Potential Link: Chronic inflammation and imbalances in gut health may contribute to the development of polyps.

14. Digestive Cancers:

• Types: Colorectal cancer, stomach cancer, etc.

• Symptoms: Vary based on the specific cancer but may include abdominal pain, changes in bowel habits, and unexplained weight loss.

• Potential Link: Chronic inflammation and other factors may contribute to the development of digestive cancers.

15. Gut Dysmotility:

• Symptoms: Altered movement of the digestive tract, leading to issues like gastroparesis or intestinal pseudo-obstruction.

• Potential Link: Disruptions in gut motility may result from imbalances in the gut nervous system.

16. Functional Gastrointestinal Disorders:

• Examples: Functional dyspepsia, functional bloating, and functional abdominal pain.

• Symptoms: Chronic or recurrent abdominal pain or discomfort without an identifiable structural or biochemical explanation.

• Potential Link: Altered gut function without clear structural abnormalities.

It's important to note that while there is a growing understanding of the gut-digestive health connection, individual responses may vary. If you are experiencing persistent or severe digestive issues, it's recommended to consult with a healthcare professional or gastroenterologist for a comprehensive evaluation and appropriate management. Addressing the underlying factors contributing to gut health may involve dietary modifications, lifestyle changes, and targeted interventions based on the specific condition.

ENTERIC NERVOUS SYSTEM

The Enteric Nervous System (ENS) is a complex network of neurons that forms an intrinsic part of the gastrointestinal (GI) tract. Often referred to as the "second brain" or the "brain in the gut," the ENS is a highly organized system that controls various aspects of digestive function independently of the central nervous system (CNS). Here are key aspects of the Enteric Nervous System:

1. Location and Structure:

• Location: The ENS is embedded in the wall of the GI tract, extending from the esophagus to the anus.

• Layers: It is organized into two main layers — the submucosal plexus (Meissner's plexus) in the submucosal layer and the myenteric plexus (Auerbach's plexus) between the longitudinal and circular muscle layers.

2. Autonomous Control: The ENS operates autonomously, meaning it can function independently of the central nervous system. However, it does receive input from and communicate with the CNS.

3. Functions of the Enteric Nervous System:

• Motor Functions: Regulates muscle contractions and movements in the GI tract, including peristalsis and segmentation.

• Secretory Functions: Controls the secretion of fluids and enzymes necessary for digestion.

• Sensory Functions: Detects changes in the environment of the GI tract, including the presence of nutrients and the mechanical stretching of the gut wall.

• Blood Flow Regulation: Influences blood flow to the GI organs.

4. Communication with the Central Nervous System: While the ENS can function independently, it communicates bidirectionally with the CNS through the sympathetic and parasympathetic branches of the autonomic nervous system.

5. Neurons and Neurotransmitters:

• The ENS contains a vast number of neurons, comparable to the number found in the spinal cord.

• Neurotransmitters, including acetylcholine, serotonin, dopamine, and others, play crucial roles in transmitting signals between enteric neurons.

6. Role in Motility: The myenteric plexus is particularly involved in regulating smooth muscle contraction, coordinating peristalsis for the movement of food along the GI tract.

7. Integration of Signals: The ENS integrates signals from various sources, including sensory inputs, mechanical stretching of the gut wall, and feedback from the gut microbiota.

8. Influence of the Gut Microbiota: Emerging research suggests that the gut microbiota can influence the development and function of the ENS, highlighting the bidirectional communication between the gut and its resident microorganisms.

9. Implications for Health: Dysfunction of the ENS has been implicated in various gastrointestinal disorders, including irritable bowel syndrome (IBS), inflammatory bowel disease (IBD), and certain motility disorders.

10. Development: The ENS develops from neural crest cells during embryonic development. Proper formation and migration of these cells are crucial for the establishment of a functional ENS.

11. Neurotransmitter Imbalances: Imbalances in neurotransmitters within the ENS have been associated with certain GI conditions, such as serotonin imbalances in irritable bowel syndrome.

12. Clinical Relevance: Understanding the ENS is clinically relevant for developing treatments for gastrointestinal

disorders. Drugs that modulate the ENS are used in managing conditions like constipation, diarrhea, and motility disorders.

The Enteric Nervous System plays a vital role in orchestrating the complex processes involved in digestion and maintaining gut homeostasis. Ongoing research continues to deepen our understanding of the intricate interactions within the ENS and its role in both normal digestive function and various gastrointestinal disorders.

IMPACT OF GUT HEALTH ON MENTAL WELL-BEING

The gut-brain connection, often referred to as the gut-brain axis, highlights the bidirectional communication between the gastrointestinal (GI) tract and the central nervous system (CNS), including the brain. This connection plays a significant role in influencing various aspects of mental well-being. Here are some key ways in which gut health can impact mental well-being:

1. Microbiome and Neurotransmitter Production: The gut microbiome, composed of trillions of microorganisms, influences the production and regulation of neurotransmitters

such as serotonin, dopamine, and gamma-aminobutyric acid (GABA). These neurotransmitters play crucial roles in mood regulation and overall mental health.

2. Serotonin Production: Approximately 90-95% of serotonin, a neurotransmitter associated with mood and well-being, is produced in the gut. The gut microbiota plays a role in serotonin synthesis, and imbalances in the microbiome can impact serotonin levels.

3. Inflammation and Mental Health: Imbalances in the gut microbiome can contribute to inflammation in the gut. Chronic inflammation, in turn, has been linked to conditions such as depression and anxiety. The gut-brain axis modulates the immune response and inflammatory processes.

4. Communication via Vagus Nerve: The vagus nerve serves as a major communication highway between the gut and the brain. Signals from the gut, including information about nutrient absorption and gut microbial activity, are transmitted to the brain through the vagus nerve.

5. Impact on Stress Response: The gut microbiota can influence the HPA (hypothalamic-pituitary-adrenal) axis, a key

component of the body's stress response system. Dysregulation in the gut-brain axis may contribute to altered stress responses and susceptibility to stress-related mental health issues.

6. Gut Hormones and Appetite Regulation: Gut hormones, such as ghrelin and leptin, not only regulate appetite and energy balance but also have effects on mood and cognitive function. Imbalances in these hormones may impact mental well-being.

7. Neurotransmitter Precursors: The gut microbiota can produce metabolites and precursor molecules that influence the synthesis of neurotransmitters. For example, certain gut bacteria can produce short-chain fatty acids (SCFAs), which may have neuroactive effects.

8. Gut Dysbiosis and Mental Health Conditions: Changes in the composition of the gut microbiome, known as gut dysbiosis, have been associated with mental health conditions such as depression, anxiety, and even neurodevelopmental disorders.

9. Effects of Antibiotics and Medications: Antibiotics and certain medications can alter the balance of the gut microbiome. Such changes may have implications for mental health, and

disruptions in the microbiome have been linked to mood disturbances.

10. Nutrient Absorption and Brain Function: The gut is responsible for absorbing nutrients crucial for brain function, including vitamins and minerals. Malabsorption or nutrient deficiencies due to gut issues can affect cognitive function and mental well-being.

11. Impact on Cognitive Function: Emerging research suggests that the gut microbiota may influence cognitive functions such as memory and learning. Alterations in the gut-brain axis could impact cognitive health.

12. Role in Neurological Disorders: Disruptions in the gut-brain axis have been explored in the context of neurodegenerative disorders such as Parkinson's and Alzheimer's diseases, emphasizing the potential link between gut health and neurological health.

13. Probiotics and Mental Health: Probiotics, which are beneficial bacteria, have been investigated for their potential to positively impact mental well-being. Some studies suggest that

certain probiotics may have a role in alleviating symptoms of depression and anxiety.

14. Effects of Diet on Gut and Mental Health: Dietary choices can influence the composition of the gut microbiome and, consequently, impact mental health. Diets rich in fiber, prebiotics, and diverse nutrients support a healthy gut and may have positive effects on mental well-being.

15. Psychobiotics: Psychobiotics refer to probiotics or prebiotics that, when ingested in adequate amounts, may have a positive impact on mental health. These include certain strains of bacteria that have been studied for their potential mental health benefits.

Understanding the intricate relationship between gut health and mental well-being provides insights into novel approaches for supporting mental health, such as personalized dietary interventions, probiotic supplementation, and lifestyle modifications. It's important to note that research in this field is ongoing, and individual responses to interventions may vary. If someone is experiencing mental health concerns, it's advisable to consult with a healthcare professional for a comprehensive evaluation and appropriate guidance.

ROLE OF GUT MICROBIOME IN NEUROLOGICAL CONDITIONS

The gut microbiome, consisting of trillions of microorganisms residing in the gastrointestinal tract, has a substantial impact on various aspects of human health, including its potential role in neurological conditions. The bidirectional communication between the gut and the brain, known as the gut-brain axis, involves intricate interactions between the gut microbiota, the nervous system, and the immune system. While research in this area is ongoing, emerging evidence suggests that the gut microbiome may influence neurological conditions in several ways. Here are key aspects of the role of the gut microbiome in neurological conditions:

1. Influence on Neurotransmitters: The gut microbiota can produce and modulate neurotransmitters such as serotonin, dopamine, and gamma-aminobutyric acid (GABA), which play crucial roles in mood regulation, cognition, and overall brain function.

2. Neuroinflammation: Imbalances in the gut microbiome may contribute to systemic inflammation and neuroinflammation.

Chronic inflammation is implicated in various neurological disorders, including Alzheimer's disease and Parkinson's disease.

3. Short-Chain Fatty Acids (SCFAs): Certain gut bacteria produce short-chain fatty acids (SCFAs) through the fermentation of dietary fibers. SCFAs have anti-inflammatory properties and may impact neurological function.

4. Blood-Brain Barrier Integrity: The gut microbiome can influence the integrity of the blood-brain barrier, a protective barrier that regulates the passage of substances between the bloodstream and the brain. Disruptions in this barrier are associated with neurological conditions.

5. Immune System Modulation: Gut microbes play a role in training and modulating the immune system. Dysregulation of the immune response may contribute to the development or progression of neuroinflammatory conditions.

6. Bacterial Metabolites: Metabolites produced by gut bacteria, such as lipopolysaccharides (LPS), may influence immune responses and contribute to inflammation. Elevated LPS levels have been observed in certain neurological disorders.

7. Synaptic Plasticity and Learning: The gut microbiome may impact synaptic plasticity, the ability of synapses to strengthen or weaken over time. Synaptic plasticity is essential for learning and memory, and alterations may be relevant to neurological conditions.

8. Neurotrophic Factors: Gut microbes may influence the production of neurotrophic factors, which support the growth, survival, and function of neurons. Changes in neurotrophic factor levels have been linked to neurodegenerative disorders.

9. Amyloid Formation in Alzheimer's Disease: Some studies suggest that alterations in the gut microbiome may influence the accumulation and deposition of beta-amyloid plaques, characteristic of Alzheimer's disease.

10. Impact on Microglia Activation: Microglia are immune cells in the brain that play a crucial role in maintaining brain health. Dysregulation of microglia activation, influenced by the gut microbiota, may contribute to neuroinflammation.

11. Role in Parkinson's Disease: Changes in the gut microbiome have been observed in individuals with Parkinson's disease.

The gut-brain axis is implicated in the spread of alpha-synuclein pathology, a hallmark of Parkinson's.

12. Gut Dysbiosis in Neurological Disorders: Dysbiosis, an imbalance in the gut microbiota, has been reported in various neurological conditions, including multiple sclerosis, autism spectrum disorder, and mood disorders.

13. Effects of Antibiotics and Medications: Antibiotics and certain medications can alter the composition of the gut microbiome, potentially impacting neurological function. This highlights the importance of considering the gut microbiome in drug-related effects on the brain.

14. Potential Therapeutic Interventions: Strategies targeting the gut microbiome, such as probiotics, prebiotics, and fecal microbiota transplantation (FMT), are being explored as potential therapeutic interventions for neurological conditions.

15. Individual Variability: The impact of the gut microbiome on neurological conditions may vary among individuals due to factors such as genetics, diet, lifestyle, and environmental influences.

While the understanding of the gut-brain axis and the role of the gut microbiome in neurological conditions is evolving, it's clear that there is a complex interplay between gut health and brain health. Ongoing research aims to elucidate the specific mechanisms involved and explore innovative therapeutic strategies that target the gut microbiome to support neurological well-being. Individuals with neurological conditions should consult with healthcare professionals for personalized advice and treatment options.

CHAPTER FOUR

MEDITERRANEAN DIET FOR THE GUT

The Mediterranean Diet is renowned for its health benefits, and it is not only beneficial for cardiovascular health but can also contribute to a healthy gut. A diet rich in diverse, plant-based foods and healthy fats characterizes the Mediterranean Diet, and these components can positively influence the gut microbiota and overall gut health. Here are key aspects of how the Mediterranean Diet can support gut health:

1. Abundance of Fruits and Vegetables:

• Benefit: Rich in fiber, vitamins, minerals, and antioxidants that promote the growth of beneficial gut bacteria.

• Recommendation: Aim for a variety of colorful fruits and vegetables daily.

2. Whole Grains:

• Benefit: Whole grains are a good source of fiber, supporting regular bowel movements and fostering a diverse gut microbiome.

• Recommendation: Choose whole grains like whole wheat, brown rice, quinoa, and oats.

3. Legumes and Beans:

• Benefit: High in fiber, plant-based proteins, and prebiotics that nourish beneficial gut bacteria.

• Recommendation: Include lentils, chickpeas, black beans, and other legumes in your meals.

4. Healthy Fats:

• Benefit: Olive oil, a staple in the Mediterranean Diet, contains monounsaturated fats that can support the gut lining and microbial diversity.

• Recommendation: Use extra virgin olive oil as your primary cooking oil and drizzle it on salads.

5. Fatty Fish:

• Benefit: Fatty fish like salmon, mackerel, and sardines are rich in omega-3 fatty acids, which have anti-inflammatory properties and may positively impact the gut.

• Recommendation: Aim for at least two servings of fatty fish per week.

6. Moderate Dairy Consumption:

• Benefit: Yogurt and other fermented dairy products contain probiotics, beneficial bacteria that support gut health.

• Recommendation: Choose plain, unsweetened yogurt with live cultures, and limit high-fat dairy.

7. Nuts and Seeds:

• Benefit: Good sources of fiber, healthy fats, and various nutrients that contribute to a healthy gut.

• Recommendation: Incorporate a variety of nuts and seeds, such as almonds, walnuts, chia seeds, and flaxseeds.

8. Herbs and Spices:

• Benefit: Many herbs and spices used in Mediterranean cuisine, such as garlic, oregano, and thyme, have antimicrobial and anti-inflammatory properties.

• Recommendation: Use a variety of herbs and spices to add flavor to your dishes.

9. Red Wine in Moderation:

• Benefit: Some studies suggest that moderate consumption of red wine may have positive effects on the gut microbiota.

• Recommendation: If you consume alcohol, do so in moderation, and choose red wine over other alcoholic beverages.

10. Hydration with Water:

• Benefit: Staying well-hydrated with water supports overall health, including digestive function.

• Recommendation: Drink plenty of water throughout the day.

11. Limit Processed Foods and Sugars:

• Benefit: Minimizing processed foods and added sugars can help maintain a healthy balance of gut bacteria.

• Recommendation: Choose whole, minimally processed foods over highly processed options.

12. Regular Physical Activity:

• Benefit: Exercise is associated with a more diverse and beneficial gut microbiota.

• Recommendation: Incorporate regular physical activity into your routine.

13. Social Aspects of Eating:

• Benefit: The Mediterranean Diet often emphasizes communal meals and a relaxed approach to dining, promoting positive mental well-being, which can indirectly impact gut health.

• Recommendation: Enjoy meals with family and friends, and savor the dining experience.

14. Intermittent Fasting:

• Benefit: Some individuals following the Mediterranean Diet may incorporate intermittent fasting, which has been associated with positive effects on the gut microbiota.

• Recommendation: If considering intermittent fasting, consult with a healthcare professional for personalized guidance.

Adopting the Mediterranean Diet is not only about individual foods but also about embracing a holistic lifestyle approach. It encourages a balance of nutrient-dense foods, social connection, and a mindful approach to eating. Keep in mind that individual responses to dietary patterns can vary, and consulting with a healthcare professional or registered dietitian can provide personalized guidance based on individual health needs and goals.

PLANT-BASED DIETS FOR THE GUT

Plant-based diets, which primarily focus on foods derived from plants and exclude or minimize animal products, have been associated with various health benefits, including improvements in gut health. Plant-based diets are rich in fiber, antioxidants, and a diverse array of nutrients, all of which contribute to a favorable environment for the gut microbiota. Here are key aspects of how plant-based diets support gut health:

1. High Fiber Content:

• Benefit: Plant-based diets are typically rich in dietary fiber, which promotes bowel regularity, supports a diverse microbiome, and produces short-chain fatty acids (SCFAs) through fermentation.

• Recommendation: Include a variety of whole plant foods like fruits, vegetables, whole grains, legumes, and nuts to increase fiber intake.

2. Prebiotics from Plant Foods:

• Benefit: Many plant foods contain prebiotics—non-digestible fibers that serve as food for beneficial gut bacteria, promoting their growth and activity.

• Recommendation: Consume prebiotic-rich foods such as garlic, onions, leeks, asparagus, bananas, and whole grains.

3. Diverse Micronutrients:

• Benefit: Plant-based diets provide a wide range of vitamins, minerals, and antioxidants that support overall health and may positively influence gut function.

• Recommendation: Eat a variety of colorful fruits and vegetables to ensure a diverse intake of nutrients.

4. Phytonutrients:

• Benefit: Plant foods contain phytonutrients with anti-inflammatory and antioxidant properties that can help maintain a healthy gut environment.

• Recommendation: Include a variety of plant foods, especially berries, leafy greens, and herbs, to maximize phytonutrient intake.

5. Reduced Saturated and Trans Fats:

• Benefit: Plant-based diets often result in lower intake of saturated and trans fats, which can positively impact cardiovascular health and may indirectly influence gut health.

• Recommendation: Choose plant-based sources of fats, such as avocados, nuts, seeds, and olive oil.

6. Probiotics from Fermented Foods:

• Benefit: Some plant-based diets incorporate fermented foods (e.g., sauerkraut, kimchi, tempeh, and certain plant-based yogurts) that contain probiotics, promoting a healthy balance of gut bacteria.

• Recommendation: Include fermented plant-based foods in your diet to introduce beneficial probiotic strains.

7. Healthy Omega-3 Fatty Acids:

• Benefit: Plant-based sources of omega-3 fatty acids, such as flaxseeds, chia seeds, and walnuts, may have anti-inflammatory effects that support gut health.

• Recommendation: Include these plant-based sources of omega-3s in your diet.

8. Reduced Red and Processed Meat:

• Benefit: Plant-based diets often limit or exclude red and processed meats, which are associated with an increased risk of certain gut-related conditions.

• Recommendation: Choose plant-based protein sources like legumes, tofu, tempeh, and plant-based protein alternatives.

9. Increased Antioxidant Intake:

• Benefit: Plant-based diets, rich in fruits, vegetables, and other plant foods, provide antioxidants that help combat oxidative stress and inflammation.

• Recommendation: Include a colorful array of fruits and vegetables to maximize antioxidant intake.

10. Improved Gut Microbiome Diversity:

• Benefit: Plant-based diets have been associated with increased microbial diversity, which is generally considered a marker of a healthy gut.

• Recommendation: Embrace a variety of plant foods to support a diverse microbiome.

11. Potential Anti-Inflammatory Effects:

• Benefit: Some plant-based foods have anti-inflammatory properties that may contribute to a reduction in inflammation within the gut.

• Recommendation: Incorporate anti-inflammatory foods like turmeric, ginger, and green leafy vegetables into your meals.

12. Alkaline-Forming Foods:

• Benefit: Many plant-based foods are alkaline-forming, which may help maintain a balanced pH level in the gut environment.

• Recommendation: Include alkaline-forming foods like leafy greens, nuts, and certain fruits in your diet.

13. Hydration with Plant-Based Beverages:

• Benefit: Plant-based diets often include hydrating beverages like water, herbal teas, and plant-based milk alternatives.

• Recommendation: Stay well-hydrated with plant-based beverage options.

14. Focus on Whole, Unprocessed Foods:

• Benefit: A plant-based diet encourages the consumption of whole, minimally processed foods, providing optimal nutrition for overall health.

• Recommendation: Choose whole foods over highly processed plant-based alternatives.

15. Balanced Macronutrients:

• Benefit: Plant-based diets can provide a balanced intake of carbohydrates, proteins, and fats, supporting overall health and gut function.

• Recommendation: Pay attention to a balanced distribution of macronutrients from plant sources.

It's important to note that individual responses to plant-based diets may vary, and consulting with a healthcare professional or a registered dietitian can help ensure that nutritional needs are met based on individual health status and goals. Additionally, plant-based diets can take various forms, including vegetarian and vegan, and individuals may choose the level of plant-based eating that aligns with their preferences and lifestyle.

IMPORTANCE OF PROBIOTICS AND FERMENTED FOODS

Probiotics and fermented foods play a crucial role in supporting gut health and overall well-being. These elements contribute to the balance and diversity of the gut microbiota, which consists of trillions of microorganisms living in the digestive tract. Here's an overview of the importance of probiotics and fermented foods:

Probiotics:

A. Definition: Probiotics are live microorganisms, mainly bacteria and yeast, that confer health benefits when consumed in adequate amounts.

B. Sources: Probiotics can be found in certain foods and dietary supplements. Common probiotic-rich foods include yogurt, kefir, sauerkraut, kimchi, miso, tempeh, and some types of pickles.

C. Importance:

• Microbial Balance: Probiotics contribute to maintaining a healthy balance of microorganisms in the gut.

- Diversity: They add to the diversity of the gut microbiota, promoting a more resilient microbial community.

- Pathogen Resistance: Probiotics may help resist the colonization of harmful pathogens in the gut.

D. Roles in Gut Health:

- Digestive Health: Probiotics support the digestion and absorption of nutrients.

- Immune System: They interact with the immune system, influencing its response and promoting a balanced immune function.

- Anti-Inflammatory Effects: Probiotics may have anti-inflammatory properties, helping to reduce inflammation in the gut.

E. Conditions and Benefits:

- Diarrhea: Probiotics can be beneficial in preventing or alleviating certain types of diarrhea, including antibiotic-associated diarrhea.

• Irritable Bowel Syndrome (IBS): Some individuals with IBS may experience symptom relief with the use of certain probiotics.

• Inflammatory Bowel Disease (IBD): Probiotics are being studied for their potential role in managing symptoms of IBD, such as Crohn's disease and ulcerative colitis.

• Individual Responses: The effectiveness of probiotics can vary among individuals, and the specific strains and dosages may influence their impact.

Fermented Foods:

• Definition: Fermented foods are products that have undergone a natural fermentation process, where microorganisms like bacteria, yeast, or molds break down food components.

• Sources: Fermented foods are diverse and include options such as:

• Yogurt: Fermented milk product containing probiotics.

• Sauerkraut: Fermented cabbage.

- Kimchi: Fermented Korean side dish, often made with cabbage and other vegetables.

- Miso: Fermented soybean paste.

- Tempeh: Fermented soy product.

- Kombucha: Fermented tea.

Importance:

- Probiotic Content: Fermented foods are natural sources of probiotics, contributing to the microbial diversity in the gut.

- Nutrient Enhancement: Fermentation can enhance the bioavailability of certain nutrients in foods.

Roles in Gut Health:

- Microbial Diversity: Fermented foods introduce beneficial bacteria to the gut, promoting microbial diversity.

- Digestive Function: Some fermented foods contain enzymes that can aid digestion.

- Nutrient Absorption: Fermentation can break down compounds that may inhibit nutrient absorption.

• Lactose Intolerance: Fermented dairy products like yogurt can be easier to digest for individuals with lactose intolerance.

• Gut Microbiome Support: Regular consumption of fermented foods can contribute to a more robust and diverse gut microbiome.

Cautions:

• Added Sugars: Some commercially available fermented foods may contain added sugars or other ingredients. Choosing minimally processed options is recommended.

• Individual Tolerance: While generally well-tolerated, individual responses to fermented foods can vary.

Incorporating a variety of probiotics and fermented foods into your diet can be a proactive step toward maintaining gut health. It's advisable to choose a diverse range of sources to ensure exposure to different strains of beneficial microorganisms. However, for those with specific health conditions or concerns, consulting with a healthcare professional or registered dietitian is recommended for personalized guidance on probiotic and fermented food consumption.

LIFESTYLE CHANGES FOR GUT HEALTH

Making lifestyle changes can significantly impact gut health, promoting a diverse and balanced microbiota, and supporting overall well-being. Here are various lifestyle changes that can contribute to improved gut health:

1. Dietary Choices:

• Fiber-Rich Foods: Include a variety of fruits, vegetables, whole grains, legumes, and nuts to increase dietary fiber, which nourishes beneficial gut bacteria.

• Prebiotics: Consume foods rich in prebiotics, such as garlic, onions, leeks, asparagus, and bananas, to promote the growth of beneficial bacteria.

• Fermented Foods: Incorporate probiotic-rich fermented foods like yogurt, kefir, sauerkraut, kimchi, miso, and tempeh into your diet.

• Limit Processed Foods: Minimize the intake of highly processed foods and added sugars, as they may negatively impact the gut microbiota.

2. Hydration:

• Adequate Water Intake: Stay well-hydrated by drinking sufficient water throughout the day, as hydration is essential for optimal digestive function.

3. Regular Physical Activity:

• Exercise: Engage in regular physical activity, as exercise has been associated with a more diverse gut microbiota and improved gut health.

4. Stress Management:

• Mind-Body Practices: Practice stress-reducing techniques such as meditation, deep breathing exercises, yoga, or mindfulness to mitigate the impact of stress on the gut.

5. Adequate Sleep:

• Consistent Sleep Schedule: Establish a regular sleep routine and aim for 7-9 hours of quality sleep per night, as adequate sleep supports overall health, including gut function.

6. Avoid Antibiotic Overuse:

• Judicious Antibiotic Use: Use antibiotics only when prescribed by a healthcare professional and complete the prescribed course. Antibiotics can disrupt the balance of gut bacteria.

7. Limit Alcohol and Tobacco:

• Moderate Alcohol Consumption: If you drink alcohol, do so in moderation, as excessive alcohol intake can negatively affect the gut.

• Quit Smoking: If you smoke, consider quitting, as smoking is associated with alterations in the gut microbiota and various health issues.

8. Proper Food Handling:

• Food Safety Practices: Follow proper food handling and hygiene practices to prevent foodborne illnesses that could disrupt gut health.

9. Probiotic and Prebiotic Supplements:

• Supplementation: Consider probiotic supplements containing beneficial bacteria strains and prebiotic supplements to support gut health. Consult with a healthcare professional before starting any supplements.

10. Diverse Dietary Patterns:

• Variety in Food Choices: Aim for a diverse range of foods to introduce different nutrients and support a broad spectrum of gut bacteria.

11. Meal Timing:

• Regular Meal Schedule: Establish regular meal times to promote a consistent feeding schedule for the gut microbiota.

12. Avoid Overuse of Disinfectants:

• Mindful Cleaning Practices: While maintaining hygiene is important, avoid excessive use of antibacterial products, as they may impact the natural microbial environment.

13. Limit Artificial Sweeteners:

• Reduced Artificial Sweetener Intake: Some studies suggest that certain artificial sweeteners may influence the gut microbiota negatively. Moderation is key.

14. Environmental Exposure:

• Nature Exposure: Spend time in nature and outdoor environments, as exposure to diverse environments may positively influence the gut microbiota.

15. Regular Health Check-ups:

• Routine Medical Visits: Schedule regular health check-ups to monitor and address any potential health issues affecting gut health.

Making these lifestyle changes collectively contributes to a holistic approach to gut health. It's important to note that individual responses to lifestyle changes can vary, and personalized recommendations from healthcare professionals or registered dietitians may be beneficial, especially for individuals with specific health concerns or conditions. Additionally, gradual and sustainable changes are more likely to be effective in the long term.

STRESS MANAGEMENT FOR GUT HEALTH

Managing stress is crucial for maintaining overall well-being, and it can have a direct impact on gut health. Chronic stress has been associated with changes in the gut microbiota, increased gut permeability, and the development or exacerbation of gastrointestinal issues. Here are stress management strategies that can positively influence gut health:

• Practice mindfulness meditation: Engage in mindfulness techniques, such as deep breathing, guided meditation, or mindful awareness, to help reduce stress levels.

• Incorporate mind-body exercises: Yoga and tai chi are forms of exercise that combine physical activity with mindful breathing, promoting relaxation and stress reduction.

• Learn progressive muscle relaxation: Progressive muscle relaxation involves systematically tensing and then relaxing different muscle groups, promoting physical and mental relaxation.

• Practice deep breathing: Techniques like diaphragmatic breathing can activate the body's relaxation response, reducing stress and tension.

• Engage in regular exercise: Physical activity, such as walking, jogging, or cycling, can help alleviate stress and positively impact gut health.

• Prioritize tasks: Effective time management can reduce feelings of overwhelm and stress. Break tasks into smaller, manageable steps.

• Build a support network: Connect with friends, family, or support groups to share feelings and experiences. Social support is crucial for emotional well-being.

• Start a journal: Write about your thoughts and feelings to express emotions and gain insight into stressors. This can help manage stress and improve emotional well-being.

• Engage in creative activities: Painting, drawing, writing, or any creative pursuit can serve as a therapeutic outlet for stress.

• Reduce caffeine intake: High levels of caffeine can contribute to increased stress and anxiety. Consider limiting consumption, especially in the evening.

• Establish a sleep routine: Prioritize good sleep hygiene by creating a relaxing bedtime routine, maintaining a consistent sleep schedule, and creating a comfortable sleep environment.

• Practice mindful eating: Pay attention to your eating habits and enjoy meals without distractions. Mindful eating can enhance digestion and reduce stress-related overeating.

• Consider therapy: Cognitive-behavioral therapy is a structured therapeutic approach that can help manage stress by addressing negative thought patterns and behaviors.

• Explore biofeedback: Biofeedback techniques can help you gain awareness and control over physiological responses to stress, such as muscle tension and heart rate.

• Spend time in nature: Spending time outdoors, whether it's a walk in the park or a hike in nature, can have a calming effect on the mind and body.

• Manage information consumption: Limit exposure to stressful news or information overload, especially before bedtime.

• Seek professional help: If stress becomes overwhelming, consider consulting with a mental health professional for guidance and support.

• Explore relaxation techniques: Techniques such as guided imagery, aromatherapy, or progressive relaxation can promote relaxation and reduce stress.

• Establish achievable goals: Set realistic expectations for yourself and break larger tasks into smaller, manageable steps.

• Find humor: Laughter can be a natural stress reliever. Engage in activities that bring joy and laughter into your life.

Implementing a combination of these stress management strategies can contribute to a more balanced and resilient response to stress, positively influencing gut health. It's important to find what works best for you, and consistency in incorporating stress management practices into your daily life is key. If stress is significantly impacting your well-being, consider seeking guidance from healthcare professionals or mental health experts.

REGULAR EXERCISES FOR GUT HEALTH

Regular exercise plays a significant role in promoting overall health, including gut health. While specific exercises directly targeting the gut may not exist, various forms of physical activity can positively influence the gut microbiota and digestive function. Here are some regular exercises that can contribute to gut health:

1. Aerobic Exercises:

• Benefits: Aerobic exercises increase heart rate and promote blood flow throughout the body, including the digestive system.

• Examples: Brisk walking, jogging, running, cycling, swimming, and aerobic dance.

2. Strength Training:

• Benefits: Strength training exercises build and maintain muscle mass, which can support overall metabolic health and contribute to better digestion.

• Examples: Weightlifting, resistance band exercises, bodyweight exercises (e.g., squats, lunges, push-ups).

3. Yoga:

• Benefits: Yoga combines physical postures with breath control and relaxation, promoting overall well-being, stress reduction, and potentially positive effects on the gut.

• Examples: Hatha yoga, vinyasa yoga, and restorative yoga.

4. Pilates:

• Benefits: Pilates focuses on core strength, flexibility, and overall body awareness, potentially supporting digestive health indirectly.

• Examples: Mat Pilates, reformer Pilates.

5. High-Intensity Interval Training (HIIT):

• Benefits: HIIT involves short bursts of intense exercise followed by periods of rest. It can enhance cardiovascular health and metabolic function.

• Examples: Sprinting intervals, circuit training.

6. Outdoor Activities:

• Benefits: Exercising outdoors exposes you to fresh air and sunlight, potentially positively impacting the gut microbiota.

• Examples: Hiking, trail running, cycling.

7. Dance:

• Benefits: Dance is a fun way to engage in physical activity, promoting cardiovascular health and overall well-being.

• Examples: Zumba, dance aerobics, salsa, hip-hop dance.

8. Mind-Body Exercises:

• Benefits: Mind-body exercises combine physical activity with mental focus, potentially influencing gut-brain interactions.

- Examples: Tai chi, qigong, mindful walking.

9. Swimming:

- Benefits: Swimming is a low-impact exercise that engages multiple muscle groups and supports cardiovascular health.

- Examples: Freestyle, breaststroke, backstroke.

10. Cycling:

- Benefits: Cycling is a low-impact aerobic exercise that can be suitable for people of various fitness levels.

- Examples: Outdoor cycling, stationary biking.

11. Stretching and Flexibility Exercises:

- Benefits: Stretching exercises enhance flexibility and can contribute to better posture and overall body function.

- Examples: Static stretching, dynamic stretching, yoga stretches.

12. Cardio Kickboxing:

• Benefits: Cardio kickboxing combines aerobic exercise with martial arts movements, offering a high-energy workout.

• Examples: Kickboxing classes, home workout videos.

13. Group Fitness Classes:

• Benefits: Participating in group fitness classes provides a social aspect to exercise and may enhance motivation.

• Examples: Spinning classes, aerobics classes, dance classes.

14. Balance and Stability Exercises:

• Benefits: Improving balance and stability through exercises can contribute to overall functional fitness.

• Examples: Bosu ball exercises, stability ball exercises, single-leg exercises.

15. Gardening:

• Benefits: Engaging in activities like gardening can be a form of low-intensity exercise and may positively influence gut health indirectly.

• Examples: Planting, weeding, digging.

Tips for Incorporating Exercise for Gut Health:

• Aim for at least 150 minutes of moderate-intensity aerobic exercise or 75 minutes of vigorous-intensity aerobic exercise per week, along with muscle-strengthening activities on two or more days per week.

• Choose activities that you enjoy, as consistency is key to long-term adherence.

• Include a mix of aerobic, strength, and flexibility exercises for overall fitness.

• Stay hydrated before, during, and after exercise to support digestive function.

• Listen to your body and gradually increase the intensity and duration of your workouts.

Remember that individual responses to exercise can vary, and it's essential to consult with a healthcare professional, especially if you have any existing health conditions or concerns. Regular physical activity, combined with a healthy diet and other lifestyle practices, can contribute to overall gut health and well-being.

COMMON MYTHS ABOUT GUT HEALTH

There are several myths and misconceptions surrounding gut health. It's important to dispel these myths to promote accurate information and guide individuals toward evidence-based practices. Here are some common myths about gut health:

1. Myth: Probiotics Are Always Beneficial for Everyone

Fact: While probiotics can have health benefits, their effects vary among individuals. The effectiveness of specific probiotic strains depends on factors such as the individual's health status, the strain of probiotic, and the purpose of supplementation.

2. Myth: Gut Health is Only About Digestion

Fact: Gut health goes beyond digestion. The gut microbiome plays a crucial role in immune function, nutrient absorption, metabolism, and even influences mental health. A healthy gut contributes to overall well-being.

3. Myth: All Bacteria in the Gut are Harmful

Fact: The gut harbors a vast array of microorganisms, including beneficial bacteria. These bacteria play essential roles in digestion, nutrient absorption, and immune function. Maintaining a balance of good and harmful bacteria is crucial for gut health.

4. Myth: Probiotics Can Replace a Healthy Diet

Fact: While probiotics can be beneficial, they should complement, not replace, a healthy and diverse diet. The foundation of gut health lies in consuming a variety of fiber-rich foods, fruits, vegetables, and whole grains.

5. Myth: Gut Health is Only Relevant to Digestive Issues

Fact: Gut health is linked to various aspects of overall health, including immune function, mental health, and inflammatory conditions. Imbalances in the gut microbiota can contribute to a range of health issues beyond digestive problems.

6. Myth: All Fiber is the Same

Fact: Different types of fiber have distinct effects on the gut microbiota. Soluble fibers, found in foods like oats and legumes, ferment in the colon and support the growth of beneficial bacteria. Insoluble fibers, found in wheat bran and vegetables, contribute to bowel regularity.

7. Myth: Gut Issues Can Only Be Addressed with Probiotics

Fact: Gut health is a holistic concept. While probiotics can be part of the strategy, lifestyle factors such as a balanced diet, regular exercise, and stress management also play crucial roles in maintaining gut health.

8. Myth: Gas Means an Unhealthy Gut

Fact: It's normal to experience some gas. The production of gas is a natural byproduct of the fermentation process in the gut. Excessive or persistent gas may be a symptom of an issue, but occasional gas is typically normal.

9. Myth: A Colon Cleanse is Necessary for Gut Health

Fact: There's little scientific evidence to support the idea that colon cleanses or detox programs are necessary for gut health. The digestive system has its own mechanisms for eliminating waste, and extreme interventions can be harmful.

10. Myth: Gluten-Free Diets Are Always Healthier for the Gut

Fact: Gluten-free diets are essential for individuals with celiac disease or gluten sensitivity. However, for those without these conditions, eliminating gluten may not confer additional health benefits and could lead to nutrient deficiencies.

11. Myth: Gut Health is Fixed and Unchangeable

Fact: The gut microbiota is dynamic and can be influenced by diet, lifestyle, and other factors. Positive changes in diet and habits can positively impact gut health over time.

12. Myth: Gut Health Is Only About What You Eat

Fact: While diet is a crucial factor, other lifestyle aspects, including stress management, sleep quality, and physical activity, also play significant roles in maintaining a healthy gut.

It's important to approach gut health with a well-rounded perspective, considering various lifestyle factors and individual needs. Consulting with healthcare professionals or registered dietitians can provide personalized guidance based on specific health conditions and goals.

CHAPTER FIVE

CHALLENGES IN MAINTAINING A HEALTHY GUT

Maintaining a healthy gut can be challenging due to various factors, including lifestyle, dietary choices, and individual health conditions. Here are some common challenges associated with gut health:

1. Poor Dietary Habits:

• Challenge: Diets high in processed foods, sugars, and low in fiber can negatively impact gut health by promoting the growth of harmful bacteria and reducing microbial diversity.

• Solution: Adopting a balanced and diverse diet rich in fiber, fruits, vegetables, and fermented foods can promote a healthy gut microbiota.

2. Lack of Dietary Fiber:

• Challenge: Insufficient intake of dietary fiber can lead to constipation, hinder the growth of beneficial bacteria, and compromise gut health.

• Solution: Include a variety of fiber-rich foods in the diet, such as whole grains, legumes, fruits, and vegetables.

3. Antibiotic Use:

• Challenge: Antibiotics can disrupt the balance of gut bacteria by killing both harmful and beneficial microbes.

• Solution: Use antibiotics judiciously and, when prescribed, consider supplementing with probiotics to support the restoration of a healthy gut microbiota.

4. Chronic Stress:

• Challenge: Chronic stress can negatively impact the gut-brain axis, leading to changes in gut motility, permeability, and microbial composition.

• Solution: Incorporate stress management techniques such as mindfulness, meditation, and regular physical activity.

5. Limited Physical Activity:

• Challenge: Sedentary lifestyles can contribute to imbalances in gut microbiota and hinder overall digestive health.

• Solution: Engage in regular physical activity, such as walking, jogging, or other forms of exercise to promote a healthy gut.

6. Inadequate Sleep:

• Challenge: Poor sleep quality or insufficient sleep can affect the gut microbiota and lead to digestive issues.

• Solution: Establish consistent sleep patterns, create a conducive sleep environment, and prioritize getting 7-9 hours of quality sleep per night.

7. Excessive Use of Antibacterial Products:

• Challenge: Excessive use of antibacterial soaps and cleaning products can disrupt the natural balance of gut bacteria.

• Solution: Practice good hygiene, but avoid unnecessary use of antibacterial products, allowing the microbiota to maintain a healthy balance.

8. Overuse of Proton Pump Inhibitors (PPIs):

• Challenge: Long-term use of PPIs, medications that reduce stomach acid, may alter the gut microbiota and affect nutrient absorption.

• Solution: Use PPIs under medical supervision and explore alternative approaches to manage acid reflux when appropriate.

9. Excessive Alcohol Consumption:

• Challenge: Excessive alcohol intake can negatively impact gut health by promoting inflammation and disrupting the gut barrier.

• Solution: Limit alcohol consumption and practice moderation for overall health, including gut health.

10. Rapid Dietary Changes:

• Challenge: Sudden and drastic changes in diet can lead to digestive discomfort and affect the gut microbiota.

• Solution: Gradually introduce dietary changes, allowing the gut microbiota to adapt to new food patterns.

11. Food Sensitivities:

• Challenge: Undiagnosed or unmanaged food sensitivities can contribute to inflammation and digestive issues.

• Solution: Identify and address food sensitivities with the guidance of healthcare professionals.

12. Microbiota Variability:

• Challenge: Factors such as age, genetics, and environmental exposures contribute to individual variability in gut microbiota.

• Solution: Focus on maintaining a diverse and balanced diet to support overall gut health, recognizing that individual microbiota composition varies.

13. Lack of Awareness:

• Challenge: Many people may not be aware of the importance of gut health or how lifestyle choices impact it.

• Solution: Increase awareness through education and access information from reputable sources to make informed choices.

14. Unmanaged Gastrointestinal Conditions:

• Challenge: Conditions such as irritable bowel syndrome (IBS) or inflammatory bowel disease (IBD) can pose challenges to maintaining gut health.

• Solution: Work with healthcare professionals to manage and address specific gastrointestinal conditions through personalized approaches.

15. Environmental Exposures:

• Challenge: Exposure to environmental toxins and pollutants can impact the gut microbiota and overall digestive health.

• Solution: Minimize exposure to environmental toxins when possible, and focus on a healthy lifestyle to support resilience.

Addressing these challenges involves adopting a holistic approach to gut health, including dietary modifications, lifestyle changes, and seeking professional guidance when needed. Developing sustainable habits over time can contribute to long-term gut health and overall well-being.

IMPACT OF MODERN DIET AND PROCESSED FOODS ON GUT HEALTH

Modern diets characterized by a high intake of processed foods can have a significant impact on gut health. The shift towards highly processed and refined foods in many contemporary diets is associated with several negative effects on the gut microbiota and overall digestive well-being. Here are key impacts:

1. Low Fiber Content:

• Issue: Processed foods often lack sufficient dietary fiber, essential for promoting a healthy gut microbiota and maintaining regular bowel movements.

• Impact: Low fiber intake can contribute to constipation, reduced microbial diversity, and hinder the growth of beneficial bacteria.

2. High in Added Sugars:

• Issue: Processed foods are often laden with added sugars, which can lead to imbalances in the gut microbiota.

• Impact: Excessive sugar consumption may promote the growth of harmful bacteria, increase inflammation, and contribute to conditions like obesity and metabolic syndrome.

3. Low in Nutrient Density:

• Issue: Many processed foods lack essential nutrients and are often energy-dense but nutrient-poor.

• Impact: Inadequate intake of vitamins, minerals, and antioxidants can compromise overall health, including the health of the gut and its microbial inhabitants.

4. High in Artificial Additives:

• Issue: Processed foods often contain artificial additives, preservatives, and emulsifiers.

• Impact: Some additives may negatively affect the gut microbiota, disrupt the gut barrier, and contribute to inflammation.

5. Unhealthy Fats:

• Issue: Processed foods may contain unhealthy fats, such as trans fats and excessive saturated fats.

• Impact: Unhealthy fats can promote inflammation and alter the composition of the gut microbiota, potentially contributing to gut-related disorders.

6. Altered Microbial Composition:

• Issue: Modern diets high in processed foods are associated with changes in the diversity and composition of the gut microbiota.

• Impact: Reduction in beneficial bacteria and an increase in potentially harmful species may influence overall gut health and contribute to conditions like dysbiosis.

7. Processed Foods and Gut Inflammation:

• Issue: Certain additives and preservatives in processed foods may trigger inflammation in the gut.

• Impact: Chronic inflammation can disrupt the gut barrier function and contribute to conditions like inflammatory bowel disease (IBD) and irritable bowel syndrome (IBS).

8. Gut Permeability:

• Issue: Diets high in processed foods may contribute to increased gut permeability (leaky gut).

• Impact: A compromised gut barrier can allow substances to enter the bloodstream, triggering immune responses and inflammation.

9. Shift in Microbial Metabolism:

• Issue: Modern diets may lead to alterations in microbial metabolism, affecting the production of short-chain fatty acids (SCFAs) and other bioactive compounds.

• Impact: Changes in microbial metabolism can influence various physiological processes, including immune function and energy regulation.

10. Reduced Diversity of Microbes:

• Issue: Diets dominated by processed foods are linked to reduced microbial diversity.

• Impact: Reduced diversity may compromise the resilience of the gut microbiota, making it more susceptible to disturbances.

11. Impact on Mental Health:

• Issue: The gut-brain axis is influenced by the gut microbiota. Poor dietary choices may impact mental health.

• Impact: Imbalances in the gut microbiota are linked to conditions like depression and anxiety.

12. Antibiotic-Like Effects:

• Issue: Some food additives may have antibiotic-like effects, affecting both harmful and beneficial bacteria.

• Impact: Disruption of the balance between good and bad bacteria may contribute to dysbiosis.

13. Potential Link to Metabolic Disorders:

• Issue: Diets high in processed foods are associated with an increased risk of metabolic disorders, including obesity and type 2 diabetes.

• Impact: These conditions may be influenced by gut microbial changes induced by processed food consumption.

14. Difficulty Digesting Certain Components:

• Issue: Processed foods may contain components that are challenging for the digestive system to process, such as artificial sweeteners or emulsifiers.

• Impact: Some individuals may experience digestive discomfort or alterations in gut function in response to these components.

15. Lack of Prebiotics:

• Issue: Processed foods typically lack prebiotic fibers, which serve as food for beneficial bacteria.

• Impact: Without prebiotics, the growth and activity of beneficial bacteria may be compromised.

16. Influence on Appetite Regulation:

• Issue: Highly processed foods may disrupt appetite regulation and contribute to overeating.

• Impact: Dysregulation of appetite may affect weight management and overall metabolic health.

Addressing the impact of modern diets and processed foods on gut health involves adopting a more whole-food-based and balanced dietary approach. Prioritizing whole, nutrient-dense foods, rich in fiber and beneficial nutrients, can positively influence the gut microbiota and support overall digestive well-being. Additionally, incorporating lifestyle practices such as regular physical activity and stress management is essential for comprehensive gut health.

IMPACT OF ANTIBIOTIC OVERUSE ON GUT HEALTH

Antibiotic overuse can have a significant impact on gut health, primarily by disrupting the balance of the gut microbiota, the community of trillions of microorganisms that inhabit the gastrointestinal tract. Here are the key impacts of antibiotic overuse on gut health:

1. Altered Microbial Diversity: Antibiotics can indiscriminately target both harmful and beneficial bacteria. This can lead to a reduction in microbial diversity, potentially compromising the resilience and functionality of the gut microbiota.

2. Dysbiosis: Antibiotic use can create a state of dysbiosis, an imbalance in the composition and function of the gut microbiota. This imbalance may favor the overgrowth of harmful bacteria and reduce the abundance of beneficial ones.

3. Selective Pressure: Antibiotics exert selective pressure on bacteria, leading to the survival of antibiotic-resistant strains. This can result in an increase in the prevalence of antibiotic-resistant bacteria within the gut.

4. Loss of Beneficial Bacteria: Beneficial bacteria, such as those involved in fermentation and the production of short-chain fatty acids (SCFAs), may be disproportionately affected by antibiotic use. This loss can impact various aspects of gut health.

5. Impact on Immune Function: The gut microbiota plays a crucial role in training and modulating the immune system. Antibiotic-induced alterations in the microbiota can affect immune function and responsiveness.

6. Increased Risk of Infections: Disruption of the normal gut microbiota can create an environment that is more susceptible to colonization by pathogenic bacteria, increasing the risk of

infections, including Clostridium difficile (C. difficile) infections.

7. Antibiotic-Associated Diarrhea (AAD): Antibiotic use is a common cause of antibiotic-associated diarrhea. It occurs due to disruptions in the gut microbiota and, in severe cases, may lead to conditions like C. difficile infection.

8. Long-Term Effects on Microbial Composition: Some studies suggest that the effects of antibiotic use on the gut microbiota may persist for an extended period, even after the completion of antibiotic treatment.

9. Metabolic Consequences: Changes in the gut microbiota composition due to antibiotic use may be associated with metabolic alterations, potentially contributing to conditions like obesity and metabolic syndrome.

10. Impact on Nutrient Absorption: The gut microbiota plays a role in nutrient metabolism and absorption. Antibiotic-induced changes may influence the efficiency of nutrient absorption in the gut.

11. Development of Antibiotic Resistance: Overuse of antibiotics contributes to the development of antibiotic-

resistant strains of bacteria. This poses a global health threat, making it challenging to treat infections with common antibiotics.

12. Compromised Gut Barrier Function: Disruption of the gut microbiota can compromise the integrity of the gut barrier, leading to increased permeability. This "leaky gut" phenomenon may allow harmful substances to enter the bloodstream, triggering inflammation.

13. Potential Impact on Mental Health: Emerging research suggests a connection between the gut microbiota and mental health. Antibiotic-induced alterations in the gut microbiota may influence mood and cognitive function.

14. Vulnerable Populations: Certain populations, such as infants, the elderly, and individuals with compromised immune systems, may be more vulnerable to the consequences of antibiotic overuse on gut health.

15. Selective Elimination of Specific Bacterial Species: Antibiotics may selectively eliminate certain bacterial species, including those associated with specific health benefits. This loss may contribute to various health issues.

16. Reduced Resistance to Pathogens: Loss of microbial diversity and beneficial bacteria may reduce the ability of the gut to resist colonization by pathogenic bacteria, making individuals more susceptible to infections.

17. Impact on Antibiotic Metabolism: The gut microbiota plays a role in metabolizing certain drugs, including antibiotics. Changes in microbial composition may affect the metabolism and efficacy of antibiotics.

18. Potential for Recurrent Infections: Disruption of the gut microbiota may increase the likelihood of recurrent infections, as the microbial community may struggle to fully recover after antibiotic exposure.

19. Delayed Recovery of Gut Microbiota: After completing a course of antibiotics, it may take time for the gut microbiota to recover. Some individuals may experience prolonged disruptions, especially if multiple courses of antibiotics are taken.

20. Need for Probiotic Supplementation: In some cases, healthcare providers may recommend probiotic

supplementation during or after antibiotic treatment to help restore a healthy balance to the gut microbiota.

Mitigating the Impact:

• Probiotic Supplementation: Under the guidance of healthcare professionals, probiotics may be recommended to help restore a healthy gut microbiota during or after antibiotic treatment.

• Prebiotic-Rich Foods: Including prebiotic-rich foods in the diet, such as garlic, onions, and bananas, can support the growth of beneficial bacteria.

• Diverse Diet: Consuming a diverse and balanced diet can contribute to the restoration of microbial diversity in the gut.

• Limiting Unnecessary Antibiotic Use: Practicing judicious and responsible use of antibiotics, including avoiding unnecessary prescriptions, is crucial to preventing overuse.

It's essential to use antibiotics responsibly, under the guidance of healthcare professionals, to minimize their impact on gut health and reduce the risk of antibiotic resistance. If someone has concerns about the impact of antibiotics on their gut health, they should consult with a healthcare provider for personalized advice and potential interventions.

ADVANCEMENTS IN MICROBIOME RESEARCH

Microbiome research has rapidly advanced in recent years, offering valuable insights into the complex and dynamic communities of microorganisms that inhabit various environments, including the human body. Here are some notable advancements in microbiome research:

1.   High-Throughput Sequencing Technologies: The development of high-throughput sequencing technologies, such as next-generation sequencing (NGS), has revolutionized microbiome research. These technologies enable the rapid and cost-effective sequencing of microbial DNA, allowing for in-depth analysis of complex microbial communities.

2. Metagenomics and Metatranscriptomics: Metagenomics involves the study of genetic material directly extracted from environmental samples, providing a comprehensive view of the entire microbial community. Metatranscriptomics extends

this approach to examine the functional activity of microbial genes by analyzing RNA transcripts.

3. Long-Read Sequencing: Long-read sequencing technologies, like PacBio and Oxford Nanopore, offer improved accuracy in assembling complex microbial genomes and capturing genomic structural variations. This is particularly valuable for studying the diversity and functional potential of microbiomes.

4. Multi-Omics Approaches: Integration of multiple omics technologies, including genomics, metagenomics, metatranscriptomics, metabolomics, and proteomics, allows researchers to comprehensively study the structure, function, and activity of microbial communities.

5. Single-Cell Sequencing: Single-cell sequencing enables the genomic analysis of individual microbial cells, providing insights into the diversity and functional potential of microorganisms within a community.

6. Spatial Profiling Techniques: Spatial profiling techniques, such as spatial transcriptomics, allow researchers to study the spatial organization of microbial communities within their host

environment, providing context to the interactions between microbes and host tissues.

7. Culturomics: Culturomics is a culture-based approach that aims to isolate and characterize previously uncultured microorganisms. This technique helps bridge the gap between culture-dependent and culture-independent methods, providing a more comprehensive understanding of microbial diversity.

8. Functional Analysis of Microbial Communities: Advances in functional genomics and bioinformatics tools enable researchers to predict and analyze the functional capabilities of microbial communities. This includes the identification of genes involved in key metabolic pathways and interactions with the host.

9. Machine Learning and Artificial Intelligence: Machine learning and artificial intelligence techniques are being applied to analyze large and complex microbiome datasets. These approaches help identify patterns, predict microbial functions, and uncover associations between microbial communities and health or disease states.

10. Gut-Brain Axis Research: The exploration of the gut-brain axis has gained prominence, revealing intricate connections between the gut microbiota and the central nervous system. Research in this area investigates how the microbiome influences brain function, behavior, and mental health.

11. Personalized Microbiome Medicine: The concept of personalized microbiome medicine is emerging, aiming to tailor interventions based on an individual's unique microbiome profile. This includes personalized dietary recommendations, probiotic treatments, and microbiome-based therapies.

12. Therapeutic Applications: Microbiome research has led to the development of microbiota-based therapeutics, such as fecal microbiota transplantation (FMT) for certain gastrointestinal conditions. Ongoing research explores the potential of targeted interventions to modulate the microbiome for therapeutic purposes.

13. Environmental Microbiome Studies: Beyond the human microbiome, there is growing interest in studying environmental microbiomes, including those in soil, water, and

air. Understanding these ecosystems contributes to broader ecological and environmental science.

14. Microbiome and Disease Associations: Advancements in microbiome research have uncovered associations between dysbiosis (microbial imbalance) and various diseases, including inflammatory bowel diseases, metabolic disorders, autoimmune conditions, and neurological disorders.

15. Global Microbiome Initiatives: Collaborative initiatives, such as the Human Microbiome Project and the Earth Microbiome Project, aim to characterize microbial communities across diverse environments, fostering a global understanding of microbiomes and their roles.

16. Microbiome Bioinformatics: Bioinformatics tools and databases dedicated to microbiome analysis have become more sophisticated, facilitating the interpretation of complex microbial data and supporting the discovery of novel microbial functions.

17. Ethical and Regulatory Considerations: As microbiome research advances, ethical considerations related to sample collection, data privacy, and responsible communication of

findings are receiving increased attention. Researchers are working to establish ethical guidelines and standards.

18. Public Microbiome Databases: The creation of public databases, such as the National Center for Biotechnology Information (NCBI) Microbiome Database, provides researchers with centralized resources for accessing and analyzing microbiome data.

19. Microbiome-Targeted Therapeutics: The development of microbiome-targeted drugs and interventions is an active area of research. These therapeutics aim to selectively modulate the microbiome to promote health or treat specific conditions.

20. Education and Public Awareness: Efforts to educate the public about the importance of the microbiome and its impact on health are increasing. Public awareness campaigns and educational initiatives aim to translate scientific findings into actionable information.

These advancements collectively contribute to a deeper understanding of the microbiome's role in health and disease, paving the way for innovative applications in medicine, agriculture, and environmental science. Continued research in this field holds the potential to unlock further insights into the intricate relationships between microorganisms and their hosts.

PERSONALIZED GUT HEALTH STRATEGIES

Personalized gut health strategies involve tailoring dietary, lifestyle, and therapeutic interventions to an individual's unique microbiome composition, health status, and specific needs. These strategies recognize the variability in the gut microbiome among individuals and aim to optimize its balance for improved overall health. Here are key components of personalized gut health strategies:

1. Microbiome Analysis:

• Assessment: Conduct microbiome analysis to understand the composition and diversity of the gut microbiota. This can involve sequencing the DNA of microbial communities present in stool samples to identify specific bacterial strains.

2. Health and Lifestyle Assessment:

• Evaluation: Assess an individual's overall health, dietary habits, lifestyle factors, and specific health goals. Consider factors such as stress levels, sleep quality, physical activity, and existing medical conditions.

3. Dietary Recommendations:

• Tailoring: Customize dietary recommendations based on the individual's microbiome profile. This may include adjusting fiber intake, incorporating prebiotic-rich foods, and identifying foods that promote the growth of beneficial bacteria.

4. Probiotics and Prebiotics:

• Selection: Choose specific probiotic strains based on their known benefits and compatibility with the individual's microbiome. Introduce prebiotic-rich foods or supplements to provide nutrients that support the growth of beneficial bacteria.

5. Personalized Nutrition Plans:

• Customization: Develop personalized nutrition plans that align with an individual's dietary preferences, restrictions, and microbiome composition. Considerations may include the balance of macronutrients, micronutrients, and the timing of meals.

6. Targeted Supplementation:

• Supplements: Consider targeted supplementation based on identified deficiencies or specific health goals. This may include vitamins, minerals, and other nutrients that support gut health.

7. Food Sensitivity Testing:

• Identification: Explore food sensitivity testing to identify specific foods that may be contributing to gut discomfort or inflammation. Elimination or moderation of problematic foods can be part of personalized strategies.

8. Stress Management:

• Incorporation: Recognize the impact of stress on gut health and incorporate stress management techniques, such as mindfulness, meditation, or yoga, tailored to an individual's preferences and lifestyle.

9. Sleep Optimization:

• Prioritization: Prioritize sleep hygiene and optimize sleep patterns. Adequate and quality sleep positively influences the gut microbiome and overall well-being.

10. Physical Activity Plans:

• Customization: Develop personalized physical activity plans based on individual preferences, fitness levels, and health goals. Regular exercise supports a diverse and healthy gut microbiome.

11. Proactive Monitoring:

• Regular Assessments: Implement regular monitoring of gut health through follow-up microbiome analyses, health assessments, and adjustments to personalized strategies based on evolving needs.

12. Therapeutic Interventions:

• Targeted Therapies: Consider therapeutic interventions, such as fecal microbiota transplantation (FMT) or specific medications, when indicated for certain conditions. These interventions should be personalized to the individual's health status and needs.

13. Behavioral Coaching:

• Guidance: Provide behavioral coaching and ongoing support to help individuals adhere to personalized gut health strategies. Addressing habits and fostering long-term lifestyle changes is crucial for sustained benefits.

14. Educational Resources:

• Informative Materials: Equip individuals with educational resources about gut health, microbiome science, and the rationale behind personalized strategies. Empowering individuals with knowledge enhances their ability to make informed choices.

15. Integration with Medical Care:

• Collaboration: Collaborate with healthcare professionals, including dietitians, nutritionists, and physicians, to ensure that personalized gut health strategies align with an individual's overall healthcare plan.

16. Adaptation to Life Changes:

• Flexibility: Recognize that personalized gut health strategies may need to be adapted over time due to changes in health status, lifestyle, or specific life events.

17. Genetic Considerations:

• Incorporate Genetic Information: Consider incorporating genetic information to identify factors that may influence an individual's response to certain dietary components or lifestyle factors.

18. Regular Follow-Ups:

• Monitoring Progress: Schedule regular follow-up assessments to monitor progress, address any challenges, and make adjustments to the personalized gut health plan as needed.

19. Community Support:

• Networking: Foster community support through group programs, forums, or networks where individuals can share experiences, tips, and encouragement related to their personalized gut health journey.

20. Continuous Learning:

• Stay Informed: Keep abreast of the latest research and advancements in microbiome science to continually refine and enhance personalized gut health strategies.

Personalized gut health strategies acknowledge the uniqueness of each individual's microbiome and health profile, promoting targeted interventions for optimal well-being. These strategies go beyond generalized recommendations and aim to provide individuals with tools and insights to make sustainable lifestyle choices that support their gut health journey.

CHAPTER SIX

INTEGRATING GUT HEALTH INTO HEALTHCARE PRACTICES

Integrating gut health into healthcare practices involves recognizing the significant impact of the gut microbiome on overall health and incorporating evidence-based approaches to assess and promote gut well-being. Here are key considerations for healthcare professionals seeking to integrate gut health into their practices:

1. Education and Awareness:

• Healthcare Provider Training: Provide education and training to healthcare professionals on the role of the gut microbiome in health and disease. This includes understanding the latest research, emerging therapies, and the importance of personalized approaches.

2. Patient Education:

• Informative Materials: Develop patient-friendly educational materials about the gut microbiome, its functions, and the relationship between gut health and overall well-being. Use visuals and simple language to enhance patient understanding.

3. Routine Assessment:

• Incorporate Screening: Integrate routine assessments of gut health into patient screenings and check-ups. This may involve asking about digestive symptoms, dietary habits, and lifestyle factors that influence gut health.

4. Microbiome Testing:

• Access to Testing: Explore the use of microbiome testing to assess the composition and diversity of the gut microbiota. Consider collaborating with laboratories that specialize in microbiome analysis.

5. Dietary Guidance:

• Nutritional Counseling: Provide personalized dietary guidance based on an individual's gut microbiome profile. Collaborate with registered dietitians to tailor nutrition plans that support gut health.

6. Probiotic and Prebiotic Recommendations:

• Evidence-Based Suggestions: Recommend probiotics and prebiotics when appropriate, based on the individual's health status and specific gut health goals. Stay informed about the latest research on probiotic strains and their potential benefits.

7. Lifestyle Modification:

• Addressing Modifiable Factors: Emphasize the importance of lifestyle factors, including physical activity, stress management, and sleep, in supporting a healthy gut microbiome. Provide guidance on incorporating these factors into daily routines.

8. Collaboration with Specialists:

• Multidisciplinary Approach: Foster collaboration with specialists such as gastroenterologists, dietitians, and mental health professionals. A multidisciplinary approach can address diverse aspects of gut health comprehensively.

9. Incorporate Gut Health in Treatment Plans:

• Personalized Interventions: Integrate gut health considerations into treatment plans for various medical conditions. This may involve customized dietary recommendations, probiotic supplementation, or other targeted interventions.

10. Gut-Related Disorders:

• Identification and Management: Improve identification and management of gut-related disorders, such as irritable bowel syndrome (IBS), inflammatory bowel disease (IBD), and other gastrointestinal conditions. Tailor treatment plans to individual needs.

11. Microbiome and Chronic Diseases:

• Linking Microbiome to Chronic Diseases: Stay informed about research linking the gut microbiome to chronic diseases such as diabetes, cardiovascular diseases, and autoimmune disorders. Consider microbiome-focused interventions in disease management.

12. Genomic and Personalized Medicine:

• Incorporate Genetic Information: Explore the integration of genomic information to understand how an individual's genetic makeup may influence responses to specific interventions targeting gut health.

13. Behavioral Medicine and Gut Health:

• Behavioral Interventions: Recognize the bidirectional relationship between mental health and the gut microbiome. Consider behavioral interventions, including mindfulness and cognitive-behavioral approaches, to support mental well-being and gut health.

14. Patient-Centered Care:

• Individualized Care Plans: Emphasize patient-centered care by tailoring interventions to individual preferences, goals, and cultural considerations. Involve patients in decision-making about their gut health.

15. Post-Antibiotic Care:

• Probiotic Recommendations: Provide guidance on post-antibiotic care, including the judicious use of probiotics to restore the gut microbiota after antibiotic treatment.

16. Pediatric Gut Health:

• Early Intervention: Recognize the importance of gut health in pediatric populations. Provide guidance to parents on promoting a healthy gut microbiome in infants and children through breastfeeding, diverse diets, and other supportive measures.

17. Continuous Professional Development:

• Stay Updated: Encourage healthcare professionals to engage in continuous professional development to stay updated on advancements in gut health research and therapeutic approaches.

18. Research and Clinical Trials:

• Engage in Research: Consider participating in or supporting research and clinical trials focused on gut health. Contributing to scientific knowledge enhances evidence-based practices.

19. Telehealth for Gut Health:

• Virtual Consultations: Utilize telehealth platforms for virtual consultations, providing accessibility to gut health advice and support, especially for individuals in remote areas.

20. Outcome Measurement:

Assessing Progress: Establish metrics for assessing patient progress in gut health. This may include symptom relief, changes in microbiome composition, and improvements in overall well-being.

Integrating gut health into healthcare practices requires a holistic approach that considers the diverse factors influencing the gut microbiome. By incorporating personalized, evidence-based interventions, healthcare professionals can contribute to improved patient outcomes and overall health. Collaboration, education, and a patient-centered approach are crucial elements of successful implementation.

REASONS TO PRIORITIZE GUT HEALTH

Prioritizing gut health is essential for overall well-being, as the gut plays a crucial role in various physiological functions. Here are compelling reasons to prioritize gut health:

• Efficient Digestion: A healthy gut is crucial for proper digestion and absorption of nutrients from the food we eat. An optimal gut environment ensures that nutrients are broken down and absorbed effectively.

• Balanced Microbiome: A diverse and balanced gut microbiome, consisting of a variety of beneficial bacteria, is associated with better overall health. These microbes contribute to digestion, nutrient absorption, and the synthesis of essential compounds.

• Gut-Immune Axis: The gut is a key player in the immune system. A well-balanced gut microbiome helps regulate immune responses, protecting against infections and promoting overall immune system function.

• Anti-inflammatory Effects: A healthy gut helps regulate inflammation. Chronic inflammation in the gut is linked to various health issues, including inflammatory bowel diseases (IBD), autoimmune conditions, and metabolic disorders.

• Vitamin and Mineral Uptake: The gut is responsible for absorbing essential vitamins and minerals. An unhealthy gut can lead to deficiencies in key nutrients, impacting overall health.

• Gut-Brain Connection: The gut and brain communicate through the gut-brain axis. A healthy gut microbiome is associated with better mental health, while disturbances in gut health are linked to conditions like depression and anxiety.

• Metabolic Regulation: The gut microbiome influences metabolism and energy balance. Imbalances in the gut microbiota have been linked to obesity and metabolic disorders.

• Reduced Risk of Chronic Diseases: Prioritizing gut health is associated with a lower risk of chronic diseases, including cardiovascular diseases, type 2 diabetes, and certain cancers.

• Circadian Rhythm Influence: The gut microbiome may influence circadian rhythms, impacting sleep-wake cycles. Prioritizing gut health can contribute to improved sleep quality.

• Endocrine System Regulation: The gut plays a role in regulating hormones. An imbalanced gut microbiome can contribute to hormonal disturbances, affecting various physiological processes.

• Metabolism of Toxins: A healthy gut contributes to the efficient metabolism and elimination of toxins from the body, supporting overall detoxification processes.

• Protection Against Pathogens: A healthy gut barrier prevents the entry of harmful substances and pathogens into the bloodstream. A compromised gut barrier can lead to systemic issues.

• Immune Tolerance: A well-functioning gut supports immune tolerance, helping prevent allergies and autoimmune reactions.

• Skin Conditions: The gut-skin axis highlights the connection between gut health and skin conditions. A healthy gut can contribute to clear and radiant skin.

• Impact on Aging Process: Prioritizing gut health may contribute to healthy aging and longevity by reducing the risk of age-related diseases and supporting overall vitality.

• Minimized Digestive Issues: A healthy gut is less likely to experience issues such as bloating, gas, constipation, or diarrhea, contributing to overall comfort.

• Support for Chronic Diseases: Prioritizing gut health can complement the management of chronic conditions such as IBD, IBS, and metabolic syndrome.

• Nutrient Utilization: A well-functioning gut ensures effective utilization of nutrients, contributing to sustained energy levels and overall vitality.

• Resilience to Stressors: A resilient gut microbiome helps the body adapt to environmental changes, stressors, and dietary variations.

• Holistic Well-Being: Prioritizing gut health contributes to a holistic sense of well-being, influencing physical, mental, and emotional aspects of life.

Prioritizing gut health is a proactive approach to promoting overall wellness. It not only addresses digestive issues but also has far-reaching effects on immune function, mental health, chronic disease prevention, and various other aspects of well-being. Adopting habits that support a healthy gut contributes to a foundation for a healthier and more vibrant life.

CONCLUSION

In conclusion, the burgeoning field of gut health has unraveled a profound interconnection between the gut microbiome and our overall well-being. The significance of maintaining a healthy gut extends far beyond digestive comfort, reaching into the realms of immunity, mental health, chronic disease prevention, and even longevity. As we delve deeper into the intricate dance between trillions of microorganisms inhabiting our gastrointestinal tract and the intricate workings of our body, the imperative to prioritize gut health becomes ever more apparent.

Understanding the pivotal role of the gut in digestion, nutrient absorption, and the regulation of the immune system underscores its status as a central hub for our physiological balance. The dynamic nature of the gut microbiome, shaped by factors like diet, lifestyle, and environmental exposures, invites us to consider personalized strategies for optimal gut well-being.

The bidirectional communication between the gut and the brain, known as the gut-brain axis, has illuminated the profound impact of gut health on mental and emotional states.

With emerging research highlighting connections to conditions ranging from mood disorders to neurological diseases, the gut emerges as a modifiable avenue for promoting mental resilience and cognitive vitality.

Moreover, the influence of the gut microbiome on our metabolic health, hormonal balance, and the prevention of chronic diseases positions it as a linchpin in holistic healthcare. Recognizing the intricate ways in which gut health touches nearly every facet of our lives calls for a paradigm shift in healthcare practices — one that integrates personalized approaches, educates both healthcare providers and the public, and fosters a proactive and preventative stance.

As we embrace the concept that nurturing the gut is not merely a dietary consideration but a cornerstone of a flourishing life, the journey toward prioritizing gut health becomes an empowering endeavor. With its profound implications for longevity, vitality, and the prevention of numerous health challenges, the call to action is clear: cultivate a resilient and diverse gut microbiome, tailor lifestyle choices to support its flourishing, and embark on a path toward enduring health and well-being. The revolution in gut health is not just a scientific frontier; it is a transformative journey towards a healthier, more vibrant future.